Acupuncture

Everything You Ever Wanted To Know

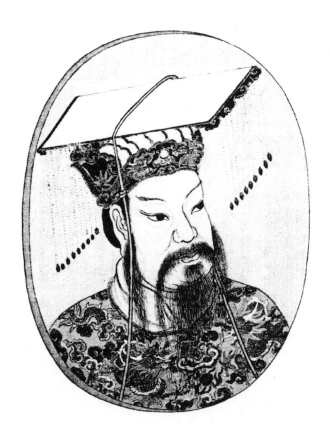

Huangdi, "The Yellow Emperor," the legendary founder of Chinese civilization

Acupuncture

Everything You Ever Wanted To Know

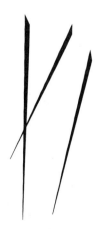

Dr. Gary F. Fleischman

Charles Stein, EDITOR

BARRYTOWN, LTD.

S

Published under the Station Hill Openings imprint of Barrytown,
Ltd., Barrytown, New York 12507. Developed in association with the
research projects of The Institute for Publishing Arts, Inc., a not-for-
profit, federally tax exempt, educational organization.

Publisher's Web: www.stationhill.org
E-mail: Publishers@stationhill.org
Author's Web: www.back2earth.com/acupuncture/

Distributed by Consortium Book Sales & Distribution, Inc.
1045 Westgate Drive, Saint Paul, MN 55114-1065.

Design by Susan Quasha and Charles Stein
Typesetting by Susan Quasha

Library of Congress Cataloging-in-Publication Data
Fleischman, Gary F.
      Acupuncture: everything you ever wanted to know / Gary
F. Fleischman
      ; cm.
      Includes bibliographical references and index.
      ISBN 1-886449-09-0
      1. Acupuncture—Popular works. 2. Acupuncture—Miscellanea.
I. Title.
RM184.F586   1998
615.8'92—dc20   95-9171
                                                      CIP

Contents

List of Questions

1 ACUPUNCTURE OVERVIEW 1
The Use of Needles 1

The Acupuncture Way of Diagnosis 7

4 CHILDREN AND ACUPUNCTURE   91

5 DIET 101

6 MEDICAL EMERGENCIES 117

7 ACUPUNCTURE AND AIDS 125

8 Cancer 137

9 Neuroligical and Emotional Disturbances 143

To my beloved parents Edward and Lillian Fleischman
whose teachings in professional dedication
and service for the public
will be with me always.

Foreword

Never before in history have so many different means of achieving and maintaining wellness been available. Technology has brought the world closer together, enabling us to draw on the wisdom of the ages from different cultures around the world. That has put into perspective the achievements, as well as the limitations, of Western medicine. Today's more informed consumers and health care providers are approaching wellness from a more self-reliant and holistic perspective.

Increased information, combined with the pending health care crisis in this country, have inspired an unprecedented interest in alternative and complementary therapies among individuals as well as health care practitioners. Encouragement has come even from the U.S. Congress, which created a forum for scientific investigation into the field in 1992, with the Office of Alternative Medicine at the National Institute of Health in Bethesda, Maryland.

What is most needed in response to this groundswell of interest and enthusiasm is for physicians with training and experience in both traditional and alternative therapies to create bridges by which interested individuals and other medical personnel can reach this great wealth of knowledge and begin to integrate the various systems to the benefit of all.

Dr. Gary Fleischman is such a physician. Traditionally trained as a Doctor of Podiatric Medicine, he has drawn on a diversity of modalities to help his patients for more than twenty-five years. This puts him in an ideal position to educate both the professional and non-professional seeker of wellness. His move to full-time acupuncturist reflects his commitment to work with the entire mind-body-nature system to restore energy, comfort and health to his patients.

Dr. Fleischman's book, *Acupuncture: Everything You Ever Wanted to Know*, fills an important void in today's health community. It provides answers to the most frequently asked questions about acupuncture and Chinese medicine, in thorough but easy-to-understand terms.

It provides an educational bridge for those curious about the uses of acupuncture for themselves, and for holistic and traditional practitioners seeking to integrate some of the wisdom of this 5000-year-old treatment modality into their own healing practices.

As founder of the International Institute of Reflexology and a practicing reflexologist for more than 50 years, I can attest to the therapeutic value of relieving blockages in energy channels. While reflexology works through different energy channels than acupuncture and involves thumb and finger pressure instead of needles to stimulate reflexes on the feet and hands, the six primary acupuncture meridians are represented in the feet. Numerous similarities between these two modalities support Dr. Fleischman's description of reflexology as a micro-acupuncture system.

The relationship between acupuncture and reflexology illustrates how practitioners in one modality can benefit from learning about other modalities. A reflexologist who understands acupuncture meridians, for instance, increases his ability to help clients with troublesome problems. In addition to working the appropriate reflexes, he can also treat the reflex areas indicated by the acupuncture meridians.

This book reflects Dr. Fleischman's traditional medical background as well as his vast understanding of the art and science of acupuncture and oriental medicine. It further reflects his recognition of our need for an informed integration of Eastern and Western therapies to ensure the health of future generations. Physicians, holistic therapists, and those interested in wellness owe it to themselves to read this book. It opens the door to a diagnostic tool, a healing therapy, a way of looking at life that leads to health and harmony.

Dwight C. Byers
President, International Institute of Reflexology
St. Petersburg, Florida

Preface

Since I began my study of acupuncture in 1972, patients and friends have continually asked me questions about China's native medicine. These questions have ranged from curiosity about the ancient Chinese philosophical outlook to practical interest in modern applications of its methods. This book is an attempt to answer the most frequently asked of these questions. I have used the question and answer format because it reflects the way in which the book arose and seemed most natural and straightforward. This format also seems particularly suited to the subject because the earliest Chinese work on acupuncture and Chinese medicine in general, *The Yellow Ermperor's Classic on Internal Medicine* (the *Nei Jing*), is presented in this way. Compiled in the later years of the first millenium B.C.E., the *Nei Jing* is, even today, the basis for Traditional Chinese Medicine. In it, a revered authority responds to questions and then adds his own commentaries. By following a similar form of presentation I hope to remove the mysteries surrounding acupuncture and help in the process of its integration with other available health services.

This process of integration will probably take some time. We are dealing with practices and ideas from two, globally separated, civilizations. Each evolved in isolation from the other over a period spanning thousands of years. The concepts and terms for understanding medical practice in the two civilizations are as diverse as their cultural outlooks and histories. It is not an easy matter to express Chinese thought in Western terms. In order to honor the integrity of the Chinese medical system and at the same time make it understandable to the Western reader, I have chosen to preserve the basic Chinese medical concepts and in some cases its vocabulary though I have attempted to explain Chinese ideas in ordinary language rather than try to find Western technical equivalents. These would often be misleading and in many cases simply do not exist. I have therefore used language intended for the lay public, rather than for either Western medical personnel or other practitioners of Oriental medicine. Nevertheless, I have not flinched from presenting the details of how diagnosis and prescription for therapy actually are arrived at. It is only through seeing how the various presenting symptoms are synthesized into a coherent clinical picture that the reader can understand how acupuncture actually helps the individual return to health.

In the process of preparing my answers to the questions on health in this book, I have had occasion to remember fondly the many physicians who have instructed me. This instruction took place first of all during my training in my former Western medical specialty, during my hospital residency. Although I made a career change to Oriental medicine, my primary exposure in patient care remains ever with me.

Teachings from a particularly eminent group of doctors practicing Oriental medicine followed my years in Western practice. Gratitude goes to Dr. Ki-Kun Wan for his thousands of hours of acupuncture training. From our professional association and friendship since 1980, I have also learned to appreciate the Chinese culture. Special thanks to Dr. Ralph Alan Dale, an outstanding instructor who explains complex Oriental procedures in plain English; and to Dr. Mark Seem, whose school, The Tri-State Institute of Traditional Chinese Acupuncture, continues to advance the profession. I also wish to thank The China Institute of Acupuncture which educates with thorough details of Chinese medical science. In addition, I cherish the valuable courses and lectures by Drs. Nguyen Van Nghi, Ted Kaptchuk, Dan Bensky, Leon Hammer, William McWilliams and Pedro Chan which I attended. Instruction from Dwight Byers in Foot Reflexology is appreciated as it coincided with all areas of my acupuncture education.

Many thanks to Charles Stein whose efforts in editing has made this book an exceptional publication. I wish to thank George Quasha for his encouragement and suggestions, and Susan Quasha for the fine art work and cover design.

I am grateful for the advice and suggestions from Drs. Bernie Siegel, Jerry Ainsworth and Ralph Alan Dale. My appreciation goes to Dwight Byers for the additional information on Reflexology. To all my patients, students and everyone else who questioned me about acupuncture, I thank you for being the inspiration of this book.

A dual medical background has made me very aware of the many ailments which are treatable by the natural routines of acupuncture but for which "high-tech" drugs and surgery offer no remedy. Yet I am aware also of the reverse situation: how the West has explored therapeutic possibilities beyond the reach of Chinese medicine. At present, many patients cannot lift their burden of affliction by any available means. Still, those who totally exclude one option over the other or settle for second opinions under the same system often limit their possibilities for recovery. All methods of health service really have so much to give us. In the end we will reap the benefits of all studies and comparisons that seek to bridge the gaps between the many forms of medical knowledge.

Introduction

Acupuncture: Everything You Ever Wanted To Know is my attempt to present the basic principles, procedures and benefits of acupuncture in a form that addresses the real questions that stand before the potential American patient of acupuncture as he or she decides whether to make use of available acupuncture services. But before we begin, it might be useful to look at the basic differences between Western medicine and acupuncture in general terms.

Acupuncture and Western medicine evaluate, prevent, and care for the same disorders but have developed historically according to very different theoretical principles and have introduced very different practical methods. For one thing, in the West, medical research has emphasized accuracy in understanding anatomical structure. This has made precision in surgery possible, encouraged the development of tools for in-depth visualization such as the microscope, the x-ray camera and MRI technology. In general, this emphasis on accuracy has contributed to the invention of innumerable precise techniques and procedures. By way of contrast, Chinese medicine in general and acupuncture in particular have always looked at how natural forces, functioning in both external and internal bodily environments, affect people. With an understanding of how blood and energy (Qi) circulate in health and disease and how changing seasonal and weather conditions may interfere with normal health, acupuncture seeks to allow the disturbed flow of blood and life-energy to return to their proper condition of harmony and balance. One might say that the West has emphasized anatomical structure, while acupuncture has concerned itself with physiology. Or again, that rather than use precise tissue analysis to aid in the development of innumerable discoveries and techniques, Chinese medicine has found innumerable ways to apply the same few but basic principles of natural existence.

The difference between the two systems shows up also in contrasting attitudes toward the use of technical instruments: the West invents and deploys many instruments to alter and correct anatomical structure, while acupuncture applies a few simple tools—acupunture needles, for instance—to correct a great many forms of physiological malfunctioning.

Physiology itself—the science of life functions—has been studied in different ways in the West and in China. European and American research explores the details of body chemistry and the activities of cells to understand processes within fluids and tissues. Chinese medicine focuses on Qi energy, various kinds of energetic polarities, circulations, climatic conditions, and the relationships between physical substances and energy. Although fluids and tissues are important in Chinese medicine, they are studied mainly for their reactions to these fundamental factors of dynamic forces.

Another difference is that Western medical science concentrates on microscopic observations of pathogenic (harmful) bacteria and viruses and seeks ways to destroy them, while acupuncture examines the afflicted bodily areas and attempts to adjust the body's systems to restore strong immunity. The pathogenic factor is understood as not only the bacterium or virus, but unbalanced aspects of the individual's total physical and emotional state, his or her personal and behaviorial habits, and climatic and seasonal factors as well. Though the details of the biochemistry of microbes may be ignored, the relationship between their activity and these more life-sustaining global conditions is attended to with extreme care.

Again, the modern, scientific disciplines which are most relevant to Western medicine are chemistry and anatomy. Chinese medicine, in so far as it seeks to incorporate Western science, is more concerned with the science that deals with energy and atmospheric conditions, i.e., physics.

Another area where the two traditions diverge is the psychological and spiritual dimensions of health care. "Mental health" as a medical category developed separately from physical medicine in the West, and ultimately became a specialization dealing with emotions, behavioral control, and abnormalities in mental functioning.

In contrast, in China, these aspects of human life were always taken into consideration as part of any acupuncture diagnosis or treatment. Emotional unbalance and behavioral or mental abnormalities were and are seen as possible causes for physical symptoms as well as symptoms in their own right resulting from energetic problems of imbalances in the Organ Qi.

Because of the general tendency in the West to compartmentalize and specialize, the spiritual or psychological aspect of physical disease is either ignored or relegated to the separate work of the clergy or the psychotherapist. Hospitals have provisions for the presence of Ministers, Priests, or Rabbis at patients' death beds, and psychological counseling may be offered to help the patient "cope" with a depressing prognosis, but there is in general no attempt to integrate treatment with the patient's spiritual or psychological state. Again, in acupuncture, anything that is of profound concern to the patient's inner life is understood to be an important factor in diagnosis and cure.

Finally, the two traditions of medicine differ greatly in regard to the historical processes by which they came into being and by which they continue to develop. The emergence of the basic principles and foundational concepts for modern Western medicine arose chiefly as a result of a continuing series of revolutionary discoveries made over the last two centuries. During the 1800s scientific researchers developed bacteriology, antiseptic technique, anesthesia, and cellular pathology. Our century has brought progress in x-ray application, antibiotics, steroid medication, and many other developments that continue to contribute to medical knowledge and practice to this day. Modern medicine is thus a fairly recent aspect of Western culture, one that coincides with the rapid development of Western science generally. Just as fundamental ideas in science are not considered absolutely fixed, so basic ideas about medicine continue to change as new discoveries are made, and even very fundamental principles are open to revision if new information, new ideas, and new methods of research seem to warrant it. But the foundations of acupuncture were laid thousands of years ago in early Chinese society, and though acupuncture itself continues to develop and discover new methods and applications, its fundamental principles have remained the same. About twenty-five hundred years ago Chinese academic medical literature began to document the basic principles of acupuncture, and, rather than alter these principles as the science accumulated more information, acupuncture developed through the steady application of them, growing and diversifying in technique and application but always remaining true to fundamental ideas. An enormous literature of such applications has accumulated over the centuries. Today, as Western science seeks by means of clinical and laboratory research to find cures for ever more illnesses, acupuncture frequently finds treatments and theoretical understanding for apparently new ailments through exploring ancient traditional medical books. (Acupuncture's way of treating AIDS is a case in point). A modern acupuncture practitioner in the West is thus much dependent on the continuing project of translating Chinese medical texts.

The answers to the questions in this book will bring to light further contrasts and comparisons between the Western and acupuncture approaches to healing.

Acupuncture: Everything You Ever wanted To Know is designed to make it easy for readers to find answers to the questions that concern them by choosing a question in the "List of Questions" and reading the answers given in the main text. Though many of the answers can be understood by themselves without further information, it will be helpful and enriching to read the introductory chapters, *Acupuncture Overview* and *The Basics of Chinese Medicine*, for a general orientation to the main ideas and terms used throughout the book. The Index should also be helpful to locate topics of interest and to help find explanations of terms not provided within each specific answer.

1

Acupuncture Overview

The Use of Needles

What does the word "acupuncture" mean?

The word "acupuncture" is a Western word, derived from the Latin, "acus," meaning "needle" and the English word, "puncture." The Chinese term "Zhue Jiao" that "acupuncture" translates really means needle *heat*, since in this form of medicine both needles and therapeutic heat from burning herbs are used to stimulate the acupuncture points.

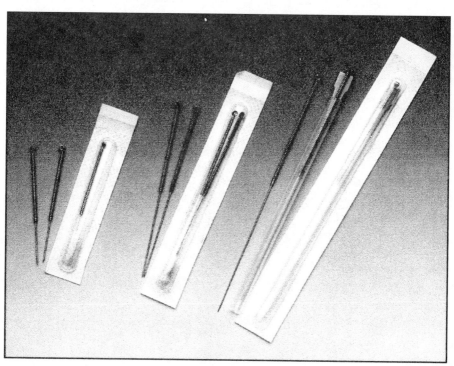

Modern disposable sterile acupuncture needles

What actually happens when an acupuncture needle is inserted?

The needle contacts and regulates an inner force called "Qi." The changes in Qi caused by inserting the needles create changes in your internal environment and restore your health. As a first step, the acupuncturist examines a system of naturally flowing Qi energies. These energies *should* function like invisible maintenance crews, whose many tasks keep the body running smoothly since Qi is behind every physiological and psychological function, from the circulation of the blood to the prevention of emotional hysteria.

If the Qi is no longer flowing well, an ailment will be in evidence. The acupuncturist then, as a second step, guides the action of the needle to return the inner workings to as normal a state as possible. Guided needles actually perform more than one hundred and fifty different kinds of healing activities, releasing blockages and restoring strength to name a few.

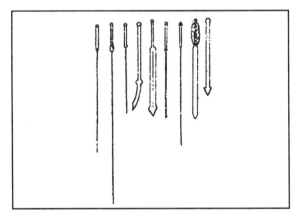

Traditional acupuncture needles

Exactly how many needles do you use to correct a problem?

The exact *number* of needles, which can be from one to twenty or even more, has some therapeutic importance. But what mainly matters is precisely *how* the needles are inserted and which acupuncture points are chosen. On evaluation of a patient's condition, the acupuncturist selects the most useful set of points to do the job. You may find changes in the locations and quantities of needles from visit to visit. Since acupuncture is very flexible, which acupuncture points are used will vary to meet the needs of the patient as different plateaus of correction are reached.

Are the needles sterile?

Acupuncture needles have no hollow shafts that might allow moisture and pathogens to gather, as can occur with hypodermic needles. Nevertheless, in Western countries acupuncturists follow strict standards of sterility. Hospitals and out-patient offices use the same methods, such as autoclave sterilization. Pre-sterile disposable needles have grown in popularity. Thus, acupuncture is a very safe procedure.

How deep do the needles go?

Acupuncturists make contact with Qi energy by inserting the needle under the skin. Certain acupuncture points involve deep insertion, from one to three inches, while some remain in superficial layers of skin. It all depends on the body part, the patient's condition, and the treatment's objectives. Needles penetrate to contact energy or, as Chinese tradition says, to obtain energy.

How long do the needles stay in?

For immediate "tonification" (the common acupuncture term for "strengthening"), a five to ten minute or quick in-and-out stimulus may suffice. Young children usually respond in a shorter period. Clearing procedures to get rid of harmful congestion take longer, possibly an hour or more. An average visit is about thirty minutes.

Do all acupuncturists treat ailments in the same manner?

Lengths of time may differ with acupuncturists, as will numbers of needles, point selection and methods of diagnosis. The many individual schools of acupuncture both in the Orient and the West have created their own methods. Initial European contacts with a single area of China gave the impression that there was but one routine of acupuncture. Now the Americanization of acupuncture combines all types of methods and techniques. We can choose from a wide range of practices.

Is there medicine on the needles?

No medicine is needed. The needle itself acts on the Qi energy to make a corrective change. Using quick or slow movements, rotations and angling, acupuncturists know exactly how to manipulate needles for the best results. There are however modern developments where medicines are deposited at acupuncture points with a needle and syringe.

How many visits are needed?

Acupuncturists tailor the number of treatments to the individual case. Everyone responds differently. Acute conditions may only warrant one or two visits. Series of six, eight, ten or more appointments may be required for persistent cases.

Do the needles hurt?

The needles usually do not hurt, except an occasional pinching sensation. Acupuncture needles are mostly thin, hair-like, solid filaments. They are not hollow hypodermic injection-type needles that can cause pain. Often acupuncture pins stimulate a pleasant sensation while the body experiences a recovery.

Will my medical insurance cover acupuncture?

Insurance companies and policies differ regarding payment for acupuncture health services. Your insurance agent can inform you of your exact coverage. Eventually, more third party health carriers will see the merits of acupuncture therapy and the cost containment that it implies.

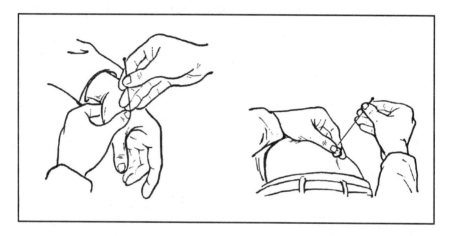

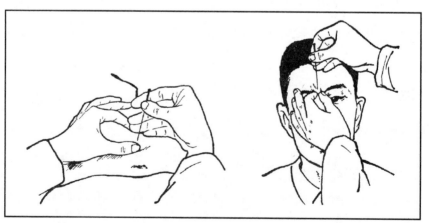

Applying Needles

The Acupuncture Way of Diagnosis

Will the acupuncturist examine my ailments differently from my own doctor, who has known me for years?

"I have an appointment with an acupuncturist because of my arthritis and poor circulation. These have never responded to conventional treatment."

Of course, acupuncture examinations will differ from your own doctor's. When acupuncturists examine patients, they bear in mind natural forces active in your external as well as in your internal environment. They also evaluate the effects these forces have upon everything else. This involves (1) examining physical body parts, (2) being aware of biochemical functions, (3) checking blood circulation, (4) inquiring as to your living habits and behavior and (5) taking into account your emotions. Most importantly, Chinese medical examinations rate the well-being of your Qi energy flow. Disorders in these forces shoulder responsibility for all uncomfortable symptoms. Irregularities in the flow of Qi energy also produce physical signs that can be recognized in your complexion, tongue color and texture, pulses and personal mannerisms. The acupuncturist puts the results of all these observations together to assess dysfunctions in the Qi energy systems.

How does acupuncture resemble traditional American medicine?

Both kinds of practitioners want to heal or at least care for your complaints to your satisfaction. Professional dedication and concern for you as a patient, desire to maintain a good reputation and desire for professional fulfillment motivate providers of health services in both traditions.

Many English language medical terms occur in both systems. For instance: "low-grade fever," "abscess," "heart palpitation." The office routines and hygienic protocols of acupuncture are similar to those learned by Western doctors. Practitioners of both traditions have been trained in schools and post-graduate programs, and both continue to keep their practice up-to-date by studying current medical journals. Both Western and Oriental practitioners are taught how to question and examine patients, and to keep records through written descriptions of the disorder. Finally, in attempting to establish a basic rapport with the patient, the two types of medicine do seem very much alike.

Is acupuncture a form of psychological treatment?

In general, no. For instance, acupuncture is not a form of hypnotic suggestion. Still, unlike Western medical practice, acupuncture does not separate our emotional from our physical well-being. In the West, mental illnesses are treated by psychiatrists and psychologists as maladies in their own right, distinct from physical problems. Western medicine has begun in recent times to study psycho-somatic phenomena, but compared to age-old acupuncture, Western research in this area is in its infancy. Chinese medicine in general is more welcoming of mind-body studies than conventional Western medicine. For a thorough analysis of the relation between psychology and Chinese medicine, I highly recommend Dr. Leon Hammer's book *Dragon Rises, Red Bird Flies*.

What are the main differences between acupuncture and Western medicine in regard to diagnosis?

Diagnoses by physicians schooled in Western medicine as compared to evaluations by practitioners trained in Traditional Chinese Medicine differ from head to toe. Western medicine knows the body by form and function, not by Qi energy. Details of a diagnosis cover cardiovascular and respiratory systems, tiny interchanges of fluids, chemical actions in cells, anatomical and physiological abnormalities, and, in general, things found to be wrong on a physical level. Doctors examine their patients with the help of a stethoscope, tongue depressor, rubber end hammer and pocket flashlight. Beyond palpating a mass, listening to sounds in the body and hammering for reflexes, diagnostic radiology and laboratory specimen technology supply a wealth of purely physical information. The outcome of such an examination results in the identification of the symptoms with a specific disease. Medicines, surgery or therapy are prescribed according to what the disease is.

An acupuncture diagnosis, on the other hand, looks for the source of these symptoms and disorders in the condition of the Qi energy as it flows or is blocked along the meridians. It often will not name and set apart the disorder as such or prescribe remedies that are associated with an isolated disease. Rather, it diagnoses the whole person and prescribes remedies designed to restore the whole being to its natural state of balance.

Without concrete knowledge of the role of bacteria and viruses in disease, how does acupuncture treat infections?

Mainly by changing the environment—inner and outer—in which pathogens (entities that cause disease) live. Infections occur where a harmful internal atmosphere and weak Qi energy cause immune deficiencies. Accordingly, acupuncture dries "internal excess dampness," removes destructive elements, strengthens Qi energy, and this improves immunity. Herbs may be needed to supplement needle treatments.

Interestingly, Western dermatologists are actually applying acupuncture principles when they treat "weeping" skin infections with a drying solution instead of with antibiotics. Many skin doctors tell about the effectiveness of clearing bacterial abscesses by just resolving moistness. From the acupuncture point of view, the viruses and bacteria are only a part of the cause of infections.

Often symptoms of infections linger after clinical evidence shows no presence of injurious microbes. These situations happen when the obnoxious guests, the germs, have left, but their necessary ambiance remains. Discouraging such "hospitality" by altering the internal environment will prevent return visits. In general, the natural elimination of pathogens by destroying their environment also has the benefit of curing symptoms without producing undesirable side-effects.

Incidentally, laboratory research on Chinese herbs demonstrates their remarkable antibacterial, antiviral, antifungal and antiparasitic properties. Unlike antibiotics, herbs do not encourage the production of resistant strains.

Should I bring X rays and lab test results to the acupuncture office?

X-ray findings and lab tests enhance clinical observations and evaluations. They may in fact prove useful to the acupuncture practitioner. However, you can only examine living Qi energy thoroughly by examining a living person. Though the acupuncturist may require such tests under some circumstances, in general, a face-to-face session with hands-on diagnostic care is the main method for coming to understanding your illness, and, therefore, your X rays and other tests may prove to be quite beside the point.

Should I tell the acupuncturist my opinion about why I am ill?

The reasons you believe to be the causes of your problems are unlikely to relate to acupuncture energy systems. However, what you actually *feel* is of utmost significance to the acupuncturist. Simply describe in full how you feel. With acupuncture, what patients *feel* is often more important than what the practitioner *sees*. The opposite holds true in Western medicine.

The acupuncturist is concerned to get a total picture of your condition. Therefore, every symptom you describe adds to his or her understanding of your disorder. In fact, the acupuncturist's examinations of your pulse, complexion and tongue are undertaken to gain further information about what your description of your complaints reveals.

My doctor has always taken my pulse and looked inside my mouth. What can the acupuncturist possibly feel and see that goes unnoticed by my doctor?

The pulse reveals much more information to an acupuncturist than it does to the Western doctor. This is because the pulse shows the state of the Qi energy systems, and these systems never entered the mainstream of Western medical knowledge.

The Western doctor takes the pulse to measure prominent physical processes and movements like the heart rate. The pulse-taking finger—in keeping with Western thought and standards—feels a *wave* in the blood stream. Heart contractions make waves, so any abnormal change in pulse rate or rhythm informs the examiner of general disturbances in heart function. Blood loss, fainting and feverish diseases also impair function and may show up on the pulse.

The pulse is also used to measure blood pressure. Causes for irregular readings—for instance, hypertension—concern the heart directly. With both pulse and blood pressure readings, the beating in the arteries is used to gain information mainly about the heart, blood volume, blood viscosity, or sometimes about a more distant kidney or liver disease.

Now in acupuncture, the sensitive fingers of the practitioner *divide* the pulse into twelve main parts, six to a wrist, that correspond to the twelve main Qi energy systems of the body. The pulse taker receives messages about living conditions from these systems. Each system is associated with one of twelve main Organs. These Organs, though called by the English names of the organs familiar from Western medicine (heart, liver, spleen, large intestine, etc.) are not limited to the physical structures and biochemical machines that we understand by them. Each organ is associated with a particular type of energy, and each energy flows mainly through a special channel called a "meridian." The meridians are named according to the Organ with which their energy is associated.

In ancient times, Chinese medical research made an amazing discovery. It found that the twelve Organs and their associated meridians interact to produce, store and trigger Qi energy. This interaction sustains and affects the entire physical and emotional makeup of a person. Since that time, diagnosis and treatment in Chinese medicine have revolved around the input and output of this system of internal Organs and its energies. The pulses serve as a valuable diagnostic tool to tell how your Organ energy is doing.

Western medical examinations may begin with looking at the tongue. Does this happen in acupuncture diagnosis too?

In Western cultures, mothers and doctors recognize peculiar changes on the tongue as signs of illness. Fever, constipation, and dehydration are known to bring out a dry and coated surface. But many other details such as cracks, colors, swellings, dots and moisture which are ignored by Western doctors are of great significance to the acupuncturist. They project a vibrant picture of the internal environment.

As with pulses, tongue examination was first used in ancient China and developed through the centuries into a precise method of examination. Diagnosis by tongue and pulse together may provide more life-giving information than X rays, blood tests, urinalysis and biopsies. When you treat *live* Qi energy, you need techniques to explore *live* Qi energy. Pictures and specimens, detached from the patient, contain no dynamic forces: the Qi energy just isn't there. All you have left is physical structure and chemistry.

Do all acupuncturists examine by pulse and tongue?

By no means. Many have developed expertise in the direct perception of a patient's Qi energy. Others may use abdominal palpation, muscle testing, observation of skin changes, and electrical or heating devices to detect problems. Those that do evaluate by pulse and tongue may not always see the need for doing so in all cases.

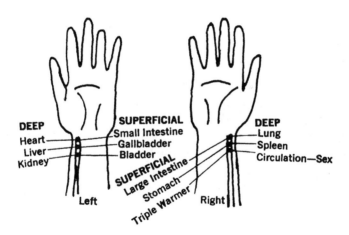

Pulse Diagnosis

Are acupuncture and Chinese medicine the same thing?

All Chinese medicine is based on the same principles that acupuncture is based on. Other techniques besides the stimulation of
the acupuncture points are often used together with acupuncture. In addition to treatment technique, acupuncture encompasses
a science of diagnosis, preventive medicine, and, as a matter of
fact, it really can involve an entire way of life. Herbal medication
evolved alongside acupuncture and often supplements needle
treatments. Other related therapies apply massage and warm
vacuum cupping over certain areas.

"Traditional Chinese Medicine," abbreviated as TCM, is generally used to designate all aspects of China's medical heritage. We
often use "acupuncture" and "Chinese medicine" as if they were
synonyms, with the awareness that Chinese medicine also includes
the intake of herbs and other therapies. Though acupuncture origi-
nated in China, neighboring countries such as Japan and Korea
learned and borrowed the basics. Just as the West took China's
discovery of gunpowder and used it to make weapons, China's
bordering nations shaped their own versions of acupuncture. We
now have the term "Oriental medicine," used largely as another
synonym, but *its* meaning really embraces all Eastern contributions.
When we mention Western medicine we mean Modern Western
Medicine. *Traditional* Western Medicine—the Western medicine of
centuries past—unlike Traditional Chinese Medicine, has little relevance today.

Can acupuncture really be used as an anesthesia for surgery?

Yes it can, though the use of acupuncture for surgical anesthesia is very recent. Electrical currents are passed through the needle to sedate an area under the influence of a specific acupuncture point. Maximum sedation brings on anesthesia.

This method has the advantage of being free from the risk of the allergic reactions associated with general and local anesthetics. With acupuncture anesthesia the patient remains awake during the operation, and all internal functions continue without interruption.

Acupuncture has been used for the reduction of pain and unpleasant sensation for at least two millennia. However, surgical acupuncture was not developed since surgery in general was not practiced very extensively in China, in spite of China's proximity to India where a complete line of corrective, surgical procedures did develop. Practitioners of Traditional Chinese Medicine limited their surgical work to draining abscesses and repairing fractures and soft-tissue injuries, including, for instance, battle wounds.

The failure to develop surgical procedures may be attributed to the strong bond that the Chinese feel with their ancestors, who brought them to this earth. Reverence for ancestry makes them feel that deceased bodies should return to the departed family intact and undisturbed. Another reason for the failure to develop surgery can be found in acupuncture theory, where it is asserted that to cut live flesh in any manner is traumatic and seriously interferes with the flow of Qi energy.

Are there any afflictions for which acupuncture should not be used as the *sole* therapy?

Many conditions do not recover with acupuncture alone. Since ancient times, China has provided necessary herbal remedies to correct ailments that acupuncture cannot heal by itself. Such ailments include diseases caused by deficiencies, infections, circulatory blockages, and those complicated by severe pain. Especially in cases of injury or illnesses where surgical repair of damaged parts of the body is required, acupuncture alone is not sufficient, though it still can be of great assistance in recovery.

Medical Practice East and West

What are some of the Western theories that attempt to explain how acupuncture works, and what is wrong with such theories?

One theory is the endorphin theory. It goes like this: The brain secretes substances called endorphins, found in the blood stream after rigorous exercise like running. Their chemical action reduces pain by blocking sensory nerve impulses. It has been found that endorphins also circulate after needling certain acupuncture points. Since the aspect of acupuncture that has been most commonly accepted by Western doctors is its power to relieve pain, it has been suggested that acupuncture works through endorphins by obstructing impulses sent through nerves. The problem is that acupuncture as practiced since the ancient Chinese is concerned with a lot more than relieving pain. Acupuncture cures and prevents diseases, it strengthens organs, balances emotions and fortifies the immune system. The release of endorphins by needling does not help to explain these by no means unimportant aspects of acupuncture.

Other attempts to explain acupuncture with Western medical concepts are equally faulty. They include relating acupuncture meridians to nerve-to-skin segments called "dermatomes" or to the autonomic nervous system. Some have even thought that acupuncture works through suggestion like hypnosis. But acupuncture needling does not depend on the "suggestibility" of the patient.

As acupuncturists in the West establish their profession and pursue further research, we will no doubt begin to develop our own way of describing the experience and effects of acupuncture. This will one day enable us to unite these points of view. For example, Chinese medical principles do deepen the meaning of the study of physiology and pathology, and this will lead one day to greater theoretical understanding. In the future it may become possible to unite the Western and Chinese theoretical perspectives, but for the time being—for the sake of good patient care and to avoid confusion—it is best if we keep concepts and theories from the two great health sciences separate.

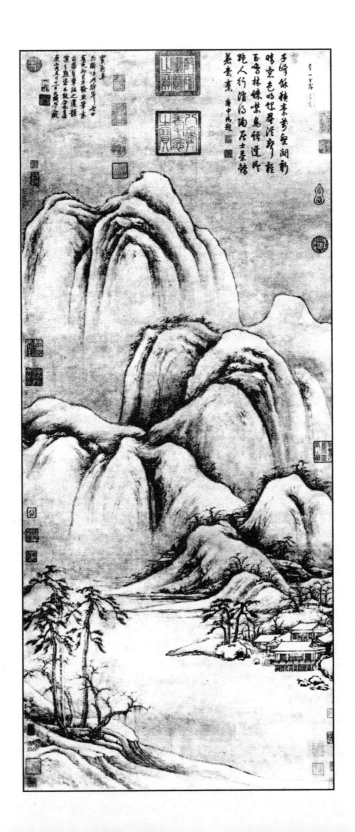

What do "allopathy" and "homeopathy" mean, and what is their relation to acupuncture?

The adjective "allopathic" comes from "allopathy." "Allos" means "other." Allopathy defines treatment that acts in *opposition* to the nature of an illness. This remains the most common approach by Western conventional medicine. With synthetic medication and surgery, doctors *fight* diseases. "Allopathy" is distinct from "Homeopathy." "Homeo" means "like" or "same." The name refers to treatments where the substances used as medicines share a nature with the disease to be cured. Instead of fighting disease, homeopathy seeks to help the body heal itself. Acupuncture is philosophically closer to homeopathy than alleopathy because acupuncture also seeks to help the body heal itself rather than fight disease.

Does specialization occur within the world of acupuncture?

Specialization as understood in Western medicine is unknown in acupuncture, primarily because the degree of interconnection between the Organ-energy systems forbids it. To limit diagnosis and treatment to one Organ contradicts a fundamental principle of Chinese medical practice, which is that all the Organ systems are interdependent. Qi energy circulates, joining the twelve Organ systems, forming a working relationship that allows one Organ to help another. A diagnosis must consider the interrelated system as a whole. Success of treatment relies on harmonizing every organ with every other.

(LEFT) *Ts'ao Chih-Po,* Mountain Peaks in Clearing after Snow. *(Dated 1350)*

Doesn't Western medicine also have a concept of balance in regard to health?

The Western concept of "homeostasis" approximates what Chinese medicine means by "balance." Homeostasis means the maintenance of equilibrium within and between the components of your body. Homeostasis is recognized by Western medicine to manage inhalation and exhalation, ingestion and elimination; new cells are understood to replace worn out retirees; hormones smoothly bring about many reactions; blood circulation easily flows to and fro. Still, homeostasis refers to *visible* activities, not the *invisible* Qi forces or the interplay of Yin and Yang, nor does it refer to the harmony between the individual and nature. It is the balance of Yin and Yang that makes up the Chinese concept of harmony, and living in harmony with nature sets guidelines for acupuncture diagnosis and treatment as it does for the traditional Chinese culture in general. Adjustments of diet, exercise, rest and all the other daily routines to seasonal and other changes, are made with a view to maintaining this balance. Thus Western medicine does have a concept that covers some aspects of balance but not others.

Western medicine fights "diseases." What in Chinese medicine corresponds to the Western concept of disease?

When symptoms have some common element or elements, Western medical science classifies them as belonging to a single disease. These elements could be a common physical organ, body system, or the fact that they are caused by a common bacterial or viral source. By examining your symptoms, physicians identify your disease. There is a hierarchy of diseases that divide ailments into groups and sub-groups according to a complex system. This is called "differential diagnosis." It differentiates between symptoms in the same group to spot the precise disease.

In contrast, in Chinese medicine there really are no differentiated diseases in the Western sense. There are names for a diagnoses such as "abdominal distension" and "heart pain," and, of greater significance, designations for different combinations of symptoms called "syndromes." These reveal underlying excesses or deficiencies of Yin or Yang energy in specific Organ systems, as well as the presence of harmful internal forces. Treatment bypasses the concept of concrete disease and goes directly to the underlying energetic imbalance.

Can you give an example of how Western medicine and Chinese medicine would diagnose the same set of symptoms?

Both methods interpret problems by drawing comparisons. Where Western doctors look for differences with similarities, Chinese medicine checks out differences with *opposites*. Take the symptoms "rheumatoid arthritis with numbness of the fingers and inflammation of the eye," for instance. The Western medical practitioner will consider a series of diseases to which these symptoms may be due. The stiff and swollen knuckles of the arthritic condition would make one suspect the connective tissue disease called *lupus erythematosus*. Widespread arthritic problems may also follow the allergic reaction of serum sickness. Numbness and eye problems are also features of sugar diabetes. We can go on and on to find diseases that share symptoms. The physician tries to find which of these "diseases" is the real culprit.

To an acupuncturist, joint pain and numbness mean blockage or deficiency, and a red eye indicates local heat caused by decreased cold Yin and increased hot Yang. The symptoms that appear on the exterior derive from interior deficiencies and disharmonies of Organ energy. The real disease itself is always the maladjusted energy.

How have the Chinese endured as one people, living on the same land and preserving largely the same culture for thousands of years?

Dr. Nguyen Van Nghi, the foremost acupuncturist in France, has pointed out that Chinese civilization has continued where other ancient civilizations have disappeared. Its survival, he said, is due to a way of thinking and a unique form of medicine.

The way that knowledge in acupuncture is deepened and widened illustrates the way that Chinese culture as a whole has been able to advance without losing its essential character. Acupuncturists do research on what is already known. Findings enrich an already established, centuries old, medical profession. In contrast, Western medicine probes the unknown. That's why our theories about health constantly change, as we forever reorganize our societies and folkways. Chinese civilization, with its medical science, remains deep-rooted and stable.

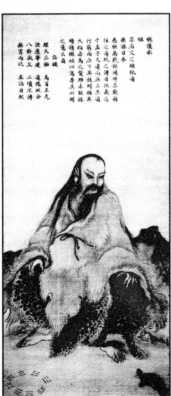

Ma Lin (Ca. 1180-1256),
Portrait of Fu Hsi

What contributions has acupuncture received from non-Chinese sources?

Answers to this question could fill a separate book. A little over a thousand years ago, Japan adopted and formed its own brand of acupuncture. In the 16th and 17th centuries, in place of the Chinese needle twisting techniques, more delicate filaments were developed to insert through a tube. Improved applications with burning herbs and expanded diagnostic routines also were developed in Japan. The book *Five Elements and Ten Stems* by Kiiko Matsumoto and Stephen Birch offers much information on the Japanese acupuncture tradition. In recent times, Dr. Kobe Akabane formulated a test to measure amounts of Qi in Organ channels by subjective means. He also invented the intradermal and press tack needles that remain in the skin for extended periods of time.

As a leader in Westernized acupuncture, France gave new meaning to old Chinese concepts. Dr. George Soulie de Morant devised a system for identifying acupuncture points with the Organ names of the channels to which they belong, and numbers to designate the specific points along the channel. Before his ingenious labeling, only Chinese adjective-noun expressions defined points. The Organ-number method has since gained widespread use. Beside this method of identifying points, other works by Dr. Soulie de Morant, and works by Drs. A. Chamfrault, Yves Requena and others have enriched acupuncture in many ways.

British research and writings (for instance, those by Dr. Felix Mann, Dr. Royston Low, Julian Scott, and Giovanni Macciola) explaining principles and applications at length, provide excellent references for English-speaking acupuncturists. Also in England, Peter Deadman edits the academically oriented *Journal of Chinese Medicine*.

In America, Dr. George Goodheart introduced chiropractic Applied Kinesiology to assess the status of channels. He showed a definite relationship between isolated muscle contractions and Qi deficiencies. Foot Reflexology is a Micro-Acupuncture system, used with finger pressure for evaluation and treatment. Dr. William Fitzgerald laid the groundwork for the method, which was developed by Eunice Ingham Stopfel. Her nephew, Dwight C. Byers, founded the International Institute of Reflexology and carries on her work to train reflexologists worldwide. Dr. Ralph Alan Dale has researched and discovered Micro-Acupuncture systems in thorough detail over the entire body. The international and highly praised *American Journal of Acupuncture*, published in California, has subscribers in over sixty countries.

Modern applications deposit medication at acupuncture points with a needle and syringe. Also, clinics in China work with injectable herbs. The future holds endless potential for developing new methods of treatment.

In the West we pay honor to Alexander Fleming, the discoverer of penicillin, and Dr. Jonas Salk for the polio vaccine, but there are many Flemings and Salks in acupuncture, from China's past and today, throughout the world.

Are there differences in medical theory and practice among Western countries that compare with the differences between the West in general and the Chinese system?

There are, surprisingly enough, many such differences. In France, for instance, due to that country's gastronomic interests, the mode of medical thinking and attention resembles the functioning of the acupuncture Liver, with its gastronomic and various additional responsibilities. Liver energy disperses congestion, stores blood and activates all Organs. There are many similarities between acupuncture's concept of the "internal environment" and what French medicine calls the *terrain*. Also, as in Chinese medicine, concern for the strength of the immune system is given more importance than the search for the presence of microorganisms.

German medicine celebrates the heart. And the German "heart" resembles the acupuncture Heart more than the American conception of the heart as a pump. China's Organ and Germany's organ propel circulation and occupy a central seat of emotion.

In America, we consider low blood pressure to be less-risky than high blood pressure, but high blood pressure by USA standards may be normal according to British medicine. In Germany, doctors frown on low blood pressure and worry about problems with the associated vascular system. Frequently, doctors prescribe special medication to invigorate circulation. There is, by the way, a class of Chinese herbs and specific needle points which, just as these medicines increase circulation, vitalize Qi and Blood.

An outstanding feature of Britain's system of health aims at moderation. As with acupuncture, a British diagnosis relies more on a physical examination than on multiple lab and x-ray tests. Less technical screening and fewer investigations for details minimize costs in the English style of socialized medicine. Allowances in assorted health services bring natural therapies to the forefront. Possibly, this tells the reason for the growth of homeopathy and acupuncture in Brittain, which are used even by the Royal Family.

Aggressive versus conservative approaches to breast cancer are prime examples of cultural difference in medical practice and attitude. America acts aggressively to conquer the disease and prevent reoccurrence. For legal purposes, medical actions attempt thoroughness. So surgeons commonly perform total mastectomies. These radical procedures are rarities in France, where the partial mastectomy has been perfected. The French rationale for minimal resection involves aesthetics and female psychology. England also favors removal of the lump but not the whole breast, for different reasons. It's easier to do and is more economical.

Interestingly, of the four countries mentioned above, Statistics show that France, with its closest resemblance to the Chinese in general approach, has the population with the greatest longevity.

Widespread uses of homeopathic remedies in Europe second a renewed and growing interest in the USA. Homeopathy is available as a post-graduate field of medicine to European doctors who regularly prescribe these highly diluted medications with success. Homeopathic remedies are available in the USA only through Homeopathic doctors and specialists in natural health.

Can the sky-rocketing costs of medical care be reduced by the introduction of Chinese medicine?

Money spent on health insurance in the United States indeed continues to skyrocket. Every year costs go up, but *conditions* of health decline, as seen by the recent spread of respiratory diseases, breast cancer and AIDS. Meantime, people want and deserve top services without emptying their pocketbooks. The enormous cost of health care has become a major issue for our government.

The solution to this problem will come from the availability of options in all forms of therapy and from an integrated health care system. Patients who pay for their insurance premiums now are forced to depend on covered services. But frequently *uncovered* services may be more effective, safer and less costly.

Ethnic diversity strengthens our country. Conversely, conflicts between cultural groups weaken American society. These principles hold true for health services. Diversified and accessible methods to care for the sick will strengthen our nation's well-being and contain costs. Sadly, the fighting within and between professions has deprived the American people of valuable therapies. Furthermore, the *suppression* that results from these battles restricts scientific knowledge that in fact could prevent and treat diseases with less expense. We're left with both limited directions for understanding wellness and sickness, and inflated doctor bills.

How have conflicts within the medical profession contributed to the cost of medical care?

The unfortunate antagonism between allopathic medical speci-alities and the natural health fields, with costly attempts by one group to discredit and suppress the other through lobbying and negative publicity, results in greater cost to the public. Chinese medicine, chiropractic, naturopathy and the health-food indus-try should not be viewed as competitors but as co-participants in the effort to provide the best possible health care.

Should Chinese medicine replace Western medicine?

One type of practice should not replace another, one should enhance another. Dedication to improvement will create new jobs in the medical field, so there is no need for Western medical pro-fessionals to fear the introduction of Chinese medicine. A wider range of treatment concepts will offer a multitude of opportuni-ties and sustain the current medical work force. Illness always needs workers.

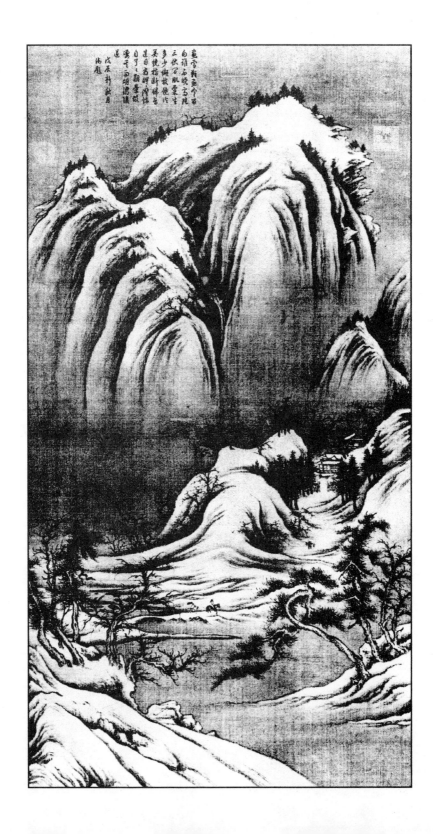

2

The Basics of Chinese Medicine

Mastering acupuncture in detail requires study and training comparable to learning microbiology, pharmacology, anatomy and surgery. Only the subject matter differs. Acupuncture makes use of Yin and Yang, Qi energy, the Five Elements, Organ energy, Channels and points. Confusion centers about Chinese medical terms. However, knowing the correct meaning of these expressions opens the door to the wondrous science of Chinese medicine.

(LEFT) *Attributed to Chü-jan,* Snow Scene. *(Undated, copy Ca. 1100)*

Yin and Yang

What are Yin and Yang?

Every aspect of existence can be understood in terms of Yin and Yang. Yin and Yang can be thought of as the two most general categories into which everything is divided. But they are not just categories: they are the basic ways in which Qi energy and everything else manifests. Yin and Yang, therefore, appear in each aspect of existence which we wish to understand. Here are some of the most important examples: In regard to temperature, cold is Yin and hot is Yang. In regard to activity, Yin is passive or receptive while Yang is active. In regard to gender, Yin is female and Yang is male. In regard to luminosity, Yin is dark and Yang is light. Again, Yang is activity, Yin is rest. These pairs of opposites always change in relation to each other, like a sea-saw: the more heat there is, the less cold, the more light, the less dark. Nothing is ever completely Yin or completely Yang. Yin and Yang mutually adjust themselves within their relationship.

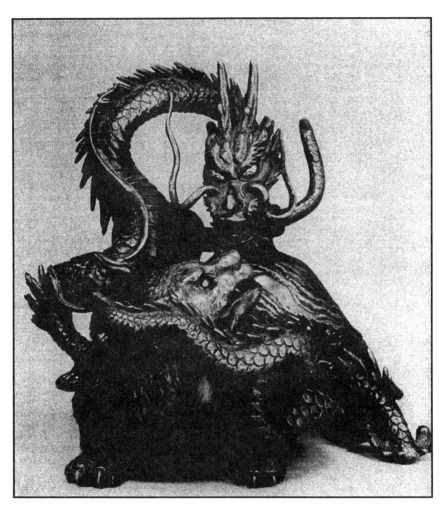

Symbols of Yin and Yang interacting through the four seasons, Japanese. (Early 19th Century)

What does "Living in harmony" mean in terms of acupuncture, and what does this have to do with "Yin and Yang"?

According to traditional Chinese thought, the purpose of culture and the purpose of existence in general is to maintain harmonious living. The purpose of acupuncture is to maintain harmony in our physical and emotional lives. The ancients saw everything in creation as a play of opposites: objects, actions, conditions, positions or potentials all exist in a process of change passing back and forth between two very general "poles" called "Yin" and "Yang." Yin and Yang are opposites, but they are not fundamentally antagonistic to each other. In fact it is by allowing the Yin and Yang in every situation to exist in harmony that the ideal of harmonious existence is achieved. Yin and Yang are thus very flexible and compatible with each other.

Living in harmony means accommodating, making room for, the interrelation of Yin and Yang within things. You balance Yang exercise with Yin rest, hot Yang summer with cold Yin drinks and cold Yin winter with hot Yang soup. Every aspect of life and existence can be seen in this way, and therefore, by balancing Yin and Yang, harmony can be brought to every aspect of existence.

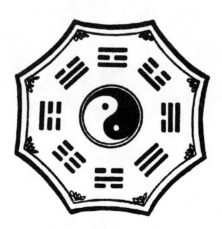

The eight trigrams of the I Ching (The Book of Changes) *surrounding the traditional symbol for Yin and Yang. This symbol is called "Tai Ch'i," the "Supreme Ultimate," because it stands for the process by which all things interact.*

How do you diagnose an illness by focusing on a Yin and Yang imbalance?

An acupuncture diagnosis takes into account many areas of imbalance and uses the concepts of Yin and Yang to understand them. The traditional system of evaluation uses "The Eight Principle Pattern" specifying four pairs of qualities or diagnostic features for examination. Each pair consists of a Yin and a Yang. Three of these pairs are hot (Yang) and cold (Yin), interior (Yin) and exterior (Yang), excess (Yang) and deficiency (Yin). The fourth pair is Yin-Yang itself and includes other general signs, such as passive (Yin) or aggressive (Yang) behavior. The diagnosis locates where Yin and Yang are in excess or deficiency and prescribes acupuncture, herbs, dietary changes, or other means to restore the balance.

What's the connection between Qi energy and Yin and Yang?

Qi energy comes in many unseen shapes and sizes, and is generally associated with the Organ-meridian systems. Qi energy is active and in constant motion and therefore has Yang qualities. With more Yang there is more energy. When there is a deficiency of Qi energy, Yin (breakdown) symptoms appear. In diagnosing the acupuncture way, Yin-Yang and Qi energy have distinct, separate functions. Qi energy is something that exists in itself. Yin-Yang is a way of characterizing polar qualitites as they are observed. Qi energy gives Organs sustenance and life. Yin and Yang serve as regulators for physiological harmony. Factors in Chinese medicine *define* one another, and yet *maintain* individual identities.

Do Yin and Yang play a part in treatment with needles?

Yes. Needles stimulate acupuncture points to restore health. The pattern of symptoms determines whether there are deficiencies in Yin or Yang that may need replenishing, or harmful excesses that must be eliminated. Needling performs these functions. Acupuncturists adjust your body the way you fine tune your television set. If you cannot hear your program, you turn up your volume. You may want to sharpen the picture, regulate the color or change the channel. The advanced technology with which you monitor your reception awaits inside your remote control and TV. Likewise, according to acupuncture theory, you have within yourself the capacity for self-healing. On occasion, you need fine tuning with needles, instead of buttons and dials.

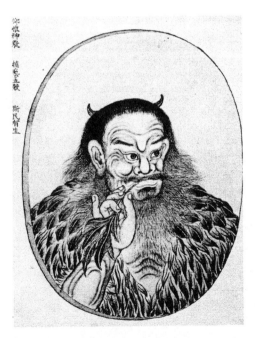

Shennong, traditional inventor of Chinese Herbal Therapy

How do Chinese herbs affect the body?

The principles of therapy that apply to needling also apply to herbology. Just as needles are applied to restore deficiencies and remove excesses, herbs are prescribed that have compensatory qualities. Herbs are characterized according to the same qualities that are found in the body, so that excess or insufficient heat or cold, for instance, can be corrected by the appropriate chilling or warming herb. The science of herbology combines ingredients to dispel harmful conditions and to strengthen weaknesses.

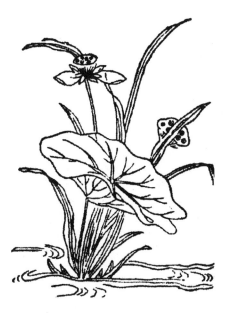

Lotus Flower (Melumbian speciosum)

In China, has herbology become a specialty like acupuncture?

It has indeed. Like acupuncture, herbology evolved from ancient wisdom into a complete medical science. Actually, the all-inclusive Chinese health tradition contains four specialized areas. These are acupuncture, herbology, massage therapy, and food therapy. Although they use different methods and materials for treatment, they overlap with similar approaches for patient-evaluation and care.

Is the worst Yin-Yang imbalance a drop in Yin or in Yang?

Neither. The *separation* of Yin and Yang that occurs under very frail conditions such as heart failure is the worst imbalance. As long as the Yin and Yang stay closely connected, acupuncture can balance abnormal states of energy. With a profound falling-out of balance, normalizing the Yin-Yang relationship is impossible. Extreme imbalance leads to death.

How are imbalances experienced in the processes of growth and aging?

At birth, Yang energy dominates. Yang fills the infant with growth potential. Young children run with endless drive. Also, we see the domination of the Yang factor in the high fever of childhood diseases. Yin takes over when we mature and, as old people, when we rest from our labors. Disorders of the young tend to be those of excess. Disorders of the elderly involve deficiencies. Excess sexual Yang energy in a young man causes nocturnal emissions and premature ejaculations. Older men experience impotence or too little Yang. To say that Yang gears you up in your youth and Yin slows you down in old age, is a good generalization of the facts. But it is also true that weaknesses (deficiencies) afflict youngsters, and, of course, society always produces a certain number of highly energized senior citizens. A Chinese rule of thumb is that we will always find some Yin in Yang, and some Yang in Yin.

How does acupuncture deal with the influence of the environment on health?

Actually, acupuncture considers two different environments: the *internal* environment and the *external* environment. One surrounds you and the other stays housed within you. Both impact upon us in profound ways: (1) The external environment consists of the atmosphere — its weather and its seasonal changes, its wind, rain, heat, coldness, dryness and dampness. (2) The internal environment consists of the functioning of our organs, body fluids, sex and reproductive functions, as well as our thoughts and emotions. Ill-effects from the outside and inside can cause bodily harm. The disorders that result show up with symptoms that are classified as stagnant, deficient or excessive. How your body handles changes in these environments brings about health and disease, sustains our life and causes our death.

Acupuncturists were actually the first environmentalists. In ancient times they studied human reactions to atmospheric changes. First hand knowledge of this kind led them to discover treatments and techniques to restore and maintain normal functioning. They recognized enough of nature's ways to create a medical science.

It is only recently in the West, that programs for the study of the external environment have blossomed across countries and been related to matters of health. But acupuncture still goes further by treating the interior of the body as an inner environment with its own climates and changes in inner weather. Our personal, inner climate and energy are major concerns for acupuncture.

Qi

What is Qi?

The corresponding English word for the Chinese word "Qi" (pronounced "chee") is "energy." Qi is an invisible, flowing force that is responsible for the characteristic functioning of the Organ-energy systems and therefore for life itself. It is also found in the natural environment as the natural force that operates as air and weather. Qi can be perceived by people trained in acupuncture and other forms of Chinese medicine and culture. It is grasped intuitively and therefore is something that is more easily experienced by people whose right brains are highly developed.

(RIGHT) *Kuo Hsi,* Early Spring. *(Dated 1072) Images in classical Chinese art depicting the elements as they appear in the countryside show the many forms Qi energy takes in nature.*

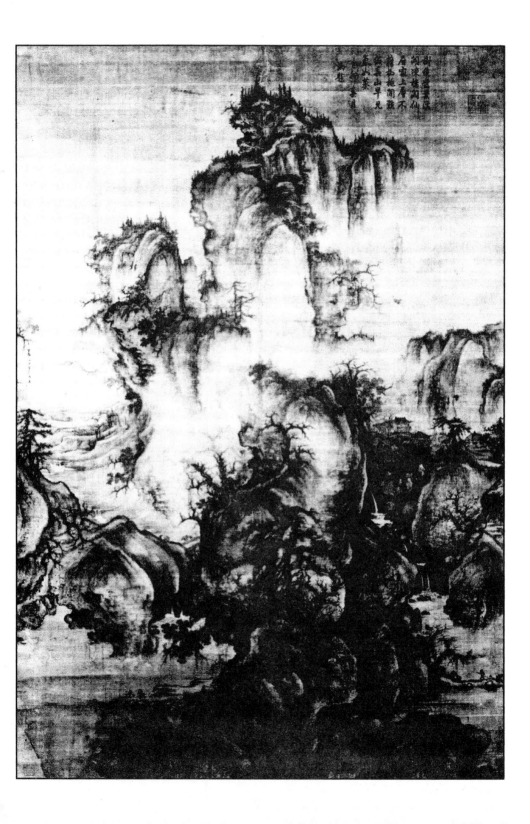

What are the different forms of Qi?

First there is Inherited Qi — the energy that we inherit from our parents. This Qi is with us at birth and is gradually used up throughout our life. When we have expended all our Qi, we die. But the original supply of Qi is supplemented by Acquired Qi absorbed from the food we eat and from the air we breathe. As a product of our Acquired Qi, another form of Qi protects us from negative factors in the environment; still another form maintains the bodily Organ systems. Nutritive Qi moves through the meridians—the channels that are associated with the twelve major Organ-systems of the body. Each energy-system has its own "flavor" of Qi. The different kinds of Organ Qi can be felt by the acupuncturist on the pulse and detected in the way the person expresses him or herself.

Where do we get Qi from?

One type we *inherit* from our parents, to last a lifetime. *Acquired* Qi comes from eating, drinking and breathing. The body transforms, transports and stores this energy, much as it metabolizes food solids. Actually, digestion is possible because of Qi. Also, we give energy to one another through acts of love and caring. The substance cannot be seen, but it can be felt. In the Chinese language, another form of "Qi" also means air and weather.

Why is the word Qi spelled with a capital q?

To recognize words in the context of their Chinese meanings, a common practice capitalizes the first letter. In discussing the kidney as an organ energy field, for example, I would write it "Kidney;" as only a physical organ, "kidney."

Is Qi the same as the electro-magnetic energy that is propagated along the nerves?

Not exactly. Qi and the "meridians" along which it moves form a system of the body never discovered as such by Western medical science. Of course Qi affects every part of you, including the nervous system. But acupuncture touches Qi energy directly. Energy then acts on selected systems, the digestive, reproductive, nervous and so on.

When faced with unfamiliar phenomena, we naturally want to compare them to something familiar. When we hear of Qi energy and the pathways or meridians along which it flows, we're inclined to think of the nervous system since it too involves energy and consists of pathways. But Qi also functions in ways that do not quite fit in with the Western anatomical and physiological picture. While Western-style research continues to try and discover what the actual relationship is between Qi and neuro-electricity, at present, most American and European acupuncture groups tend to work with the original Chinese concepts of Qi energy systems, understood according to centuries of Chinese medical research and documentation. For the time being anyway, Qi is Qi and nerves are nerves.

The Organs

What's the difference between the Western and the Chinese medical conception of the organs?

Western medicine understands an organ as a part of the physical body that performs particular functions. The liver, heart and kidneys fit this description, as well as the hand and the skin. By and large, the Chinese system refers to the same physical organs and understands many of the same functions. The Chinese system, however, includes the functioning of the specific forms of Qi energy associated with each organ, and has a very different way of thinking about the interrelations between the organs. The Chinese concept of the Organ, for instance, includes the meridians or energy pathways along which the organ Qi flows, as well as the particular emotions associated with the Organs. The different Organ-energy systems serve to support, nourish and control each other.

A work that his been very important for relating Western concepts to Chinese medicine, *The Theoretical Foundations of Chinese Medicine* by Manfred Porkert, discusses each organ as an "orb" or sphere. The different spheres of activity of the Organs interact to sustain the individual. The Qi energy from each Organ specializes in certain actions. Lung energy, for instance, functions differently from the Spleen's energy.

In brief, acupuncture manages Organ Qi, while Western medicine examines and manipulates organ structure and chemistry. Acupuncture does affect structure and chemistry but by managing Qi.

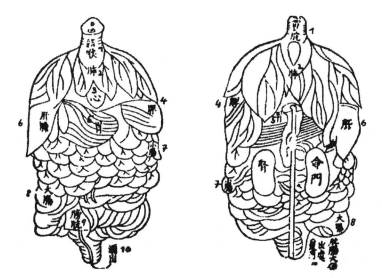

Traditional images for internal organs

In the Chinese system, how many Organs are there and what are they?

There are twelve: Lung, Large Intestine, Stomach, Spleen, Heart, Small Intestine, Urinary Bladder, Kidney, Pericardium, Triple Warmer, Gallbladder and Liver. The Triple Warmer, called also the Triple Heater or Triple Burner, is not a single Organ, but represents the Qi energy associated with three functional areas, the upper, middle, and lower portions of the torso.

How do you know which Organ or Organ system in particular is out of order?

Primarily by examining the tongue, the pulses, the complexion, behavior and other signs such as the sound of a cough. Your acupuncturist also learns a lot through your description of how you feel. Particular symptoms indicate dysfunctions of particular Organs. Combinations of symptoms form patterns that the acupuncturist is trained to recognize. For instance, a pattern that includes dizziness, blurred vision, anger, pain in the ribs, neuro-muscular disorders and stagnating congestion, suggests a problem with the Liver. Patterns of symptoms may also suggest patterns of dysfunction among the Organs. When the acupuncturist takes into consideration all the signs and all your complaints, he or she can identify regions of internal disharmony.

In what way can one Organ help another to correct a problem?

After an examination locates the trouble in a particular Organ or pattern of Organ-energy systems, the practitioner plans his treatment from an assortment of available methods. The Organ systems are connected to each other in well-known ways. For instance, each Organ system has the capacity to supply energy to another specific Organ system. Acupuncture calls the donor Organ "the mother" and the recipient, "the child." Acupuncturists are trained in understanding the details of this and other patterns of energy transfer and control. Analyses of how these patterns apply to the patient's symptoms help them to decide which acupuncture points along which Organ-associated meridians should be stimulated by needling or other means.

Where is the Organ Qi energy located in relation to the physical organ?

The energy is located in the physical organ's vicinity, but it also projects through the meridians associated with the Organs and throughout the body.

The Five Elements

What are The Five Elements?

The Western medical tradition, before the advent of modern science and modern medicine, empolyed a four element system as the basis of its theory of the nature of the material world. The elements were fire, water, air and earth. Traditional Chinese medicine uses a slightly different, Five-Element system. This is derived originally from the ancient Chinese philosophical faith of Taoism which taught the Divine Way or Tao, with awareness of Yin and Yang and The Five Elements. These fundamental teachings entered Chinese medicine. The Elements are: Wood, Fire, Earth, Metal, and Water. The Elements are understood as "generating" and "controlling" each other, and are usually shown diagramatically arranged around a circle in two different ways, illustrating these two "cycles" of interaction. Acupuncture usually makes use of the corresponding term, "Five Phases" to define the functional nature of the pattern in transformations and ongoing cyclic repetitions.

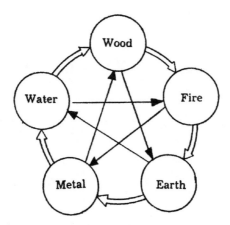

The Cycle of Generation (empty arrows) and the Cycle of Control (dark-pointed arrows). In Traditional Chinese Medicine the Five Elements "generate" and "control" each other according to the pattern in the diagram.

FIVE ELEMENT CORRESPONDENCE CHARTS
(see following two pages)

The Elements are five very broad categories for organizing phenomena both within the body and within nature. Thus, every Organ is associated with an element, and a form of sense perception is also assigned to each one; so are the different flavors of food, the different emotions, as well as the seasons of the year.The elements, in fact, reflect all apsects of existence, not only what we would call natural phenomena. Here is a chart giving many categories whose members are distributed according to the five Elements. Some groupings are obvious and some need a little imagination. Regardless, traditional China saw all of existence constructed on the same eternally functioning pattern. In our sections below on specific syndromes and diseases, we discuss the particulars of certain of these sets of five.

Five Element Correspondence Charts

	WOOD	FIRE	EARTH	METAL	WATER
SEASON	Spring	Summer	Late Summer	Autumn	Winter
ORGAN-YIN YANG	Liver Gallbladder	Heart /Peri-cardium (Yin); Small Intestine and Triple Warmer (Yang)	Spleen Stomach	Lungs Large Intestines	Kidney Urinary Bladder
TIME OF DAY	11 PM-3 AM	11 AM-3 PM 7 PM-11 PM	7 AM-11 AM	3 AM-7AM	3 PM-7 PM
DIRECTION	East	South	Center	West	North
FLAVOR	Sour	Bitter	Sweet	Spicy	Salty
ORIFICE	Eyes	Tongue	Mouth	Nose	Ears
SENSE OR FUNCTION	Sight	Speech	Touch	Smell	Hearing
SECRETION	Bile/Tears	Blood/Sweat	Lymph/Saliva	Mucus	Semen/Spinal fluid
SOUND OF VOICE	Shouting	Laughter	Singing	Weeping	Groaning
PART OF BODY	Tendons/Mus-cles	Blood vessels	Large muscles and limbs	Skin/Hair	Bone/Teeth
POWER	Birth	Maturation	Decrease	Balance	Emphasize
SCENT	Sour	Burnt	Sweet	Pungent	Putrid
CLIMATE	Windy	Hot	Damp	Dry	Cold

FIVE ELEMENT CORRESPONDENCE CHARTS (con't)

	WOOD	FIRE	EARTH	METAL	WATER
LIFE'S ASPECTS	Germination	Growth	Transformation	Reaping	Storing
DREAMS	of trees or hostilities	of laughter, fear, or fire	of being overweight, of starvation, construction, music, hills, or marshes	of white or metalic objects, murder, fright or flying	of water, boats, swimming
GRAIN	Wheat	Millet	Rye	Rice	Barley
FRUIT	Plum	Apricot	Date	Peach	Chestnut
MEAT	Chicken	Lamb	Beef	Horse	Pig
VEGETABLE	Leek	Shallot	Hollyhock	Scallions	Beans
NUMBER	8	7	5	9	6
MUSICAL NOTE	Mi	Sol	Do	Re	La
COLOR	Green	Red	Yellow	White	Black
SPIRITUAL DIMENSION	Soul	Mind Spirit	Thought	Body or animal spirit	Will
NEG. EMOTION	Anger	Hysteria	Worry	Sadness	Fear
POS. EMOTION	Assertiveness	Joy	Concern	Empathy	Courage
ACTIVITY	Walking	Watching	Sitting	Lying down	Standing
EXTERNAL STRUCTURE	Nails	Facial complexion	Lips	Skin and body hair	Head hair

What do the Five Elements have to do with acupuncture?

Each Element is represented by two Organs, one Yin and one Yang. The Elements are conceived as influencing each other in a well-defined integration: each Element is said to "nourish" one other element; each element is said to "control" one other element. There are thus two traditional patterns or cycles in which the elements are related, a "nourishment cycle" and a "control cycle" *(See the chart on page 50)*. The way the Elements nourish and control each other corresponds to the way the Organs that correspond to them also nourish and control each other. Elements can thus serve as guides for understanding the flow of Qi energy. For instance, Water "controls" the Element Fire. The Kidney is associated with Water, and the Heart is associated with Fire; therefore, herbs and needling chosen to strengthen the Kidney might be employed to reduce the "Fire" involved in very rapid heart palpitations. Many examples of the way this system works appear throughout this book.

As a standard of reference, the tables of relations among the Organ systems and Five Elements resemble the tables of norms which Western physicians use to interpret their lab test results. One deals with biochemistry and tissue, the other with energy.

What makes a Yin Organ Yin and a Yang Organ Yang?

Yin Organs exist more internally and appear to be more solid, as compared to the more external and hollow Yang. But each Organ—whether in comparison to other Organs or by its own traits—is categorized as Yin or Yang, yet has both a Yin and Yang aspect in regard to its own functioning. For instance, the Yin aspect of the Liver stores blood, while its Yang aspect controls muscles, tendons, and ligaments.

The organs are also grouped in complementary pairs, one Yin and one Yang and, as a pair, associated with the Elements *(See the chart on pages 52-53).*

The Meridians and Channels

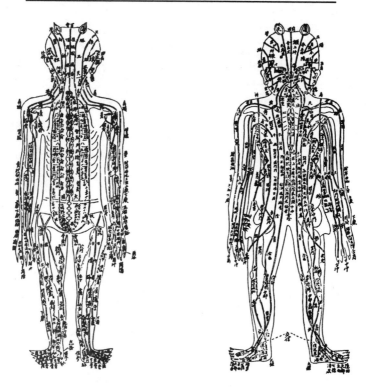

Ancient Acupuncture Chart (rear and front views)

What are the Meridians and Channels?

Qi travels throughout the body, flowing in and out of the physical Organs and up and down the head, trunk, arms and legs. A network of pathways provides the routes along which the Qi energy flows. In the early years of the practice of acupuncture in the West, English-speaking acupuncturists called these pathways "meridians," thinking of the lines that encircle a globe. However, since Qi has a depth dimension as well as the linearity suggested by "meridian," the terms "channel" and "vessel" have gained acceptance as well. Meridians, channels and vessels all refer to the pathways that direct Qi energy.

What is the connection between the Channels and the Organs?

The twelve channels are known by the names of the twelve Organs through which they pass to receive Qi energy from the source. Each channel either begins or ends at a finger or a toe. The Organ's Qi rides its pathway. As the Organs are coupled in Yin-Yang pairs, the channels connecting them are paired also, allowing the Qi energy to flow in a circular movement between the paired Organs.

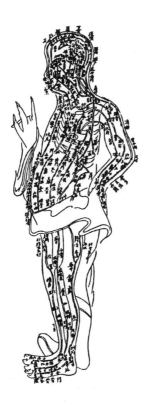

Ancient Acupuncture Chart
(side view)

How complex is the network of Channels? Are the twelve Channels associated with the Organs all that there is to it?

The system of Organ-energy channels is as complex as the physical systems of nerves and blood vessels known to Western medicine. In addition to the twelve Organ channels that connect with one another and to their Yin or Yang Organs and their Yang or Yin counterparts, there are Eight Extra meridians that stock Inherited Qi (the Qi we inherit from our parents at birth) and a group of special pathways that extends to the tendons and muscles. Junctions, side routes, rotaries, exits, entrances, descents and elevations supplement and complete the Qi energy courses. There are also minute sets of vessels that interact with micro-acupuncture systems — regions that reproduce the entire body's energy system in miniature. Such systems are recognized, for example, in the ear, hand, and, foot; and there are special acupuncture techniques that make use of these micro-systems.

What is the relation between Qi energy and disease?

Qi energy flows smoothly everywhere in a healthy person's body. When Qi ceases to flow by becoming stagnant because it is blocked or depleted, or when it is stirred up because it is afflicted with excesses, disease occurs.

How is the Chinese concept of the blood different from that of Western medicine?

The concept of blood as a bodily substance is the same in both systems. In Chinese medicine, however, the Blood is understood as working together with Qi energy. Blood and Qi move together as traveling companions. Considered as a pair, Qi is Yang and Blood is Yin. Yang Qi motivates Blood and Blood provides a medium for the movement of Qi energy. This relationship only exists in the Blood when it is functioning as part of the living organism. If you draw a specimen of blood from an artery or vein to analyze it chemically, the propulsive drive of the Yang Qi factor vanishes.

Incidentally, Chinese medicine has known about the circulation of the blood for thousands of years. The West had to wait until the seventeenth century for this knowledge when Dr. William Harvey of England announced that blood moves through vessels.

When you improve a condition with a better flow of Qi, are you also bringing in a better flow of Blood?

Exactly. Blood in acupuncture means *energized* Blood. For poor circulation and vascular diseases, treatment aims at awakening Yang Qi, which in turn increases the flow of Blood, its Yin, fluid partner (see previous question). When you improve the flow of Qi, problems caused by a Deficiency are resolved because of the increased availability of energy, and the increased flow of Blood that comes along with increased flow of Qi energy nourishes the tissues.

What gave the early acupuncturists the ability to search along the invisible meridians to find the acupuncture points?

In the pre-historic, early days of acupuncture, awareness of meridians grew from knowledge of nature's flow of action in cyclic patterns. It was observed that energy flowed in the body along certain pathways, and that there were certain points along these pathways that, if stimulated, could be used to influence the energy flow. Specific therapeutic techniques were developed through the observation of responses to such stimulation. As time went on, research and documentation lead to the establishment of Chinese medical science. The process goes on today, as acupuncturists continue to find additional points.

How does the acupuncturist know exactly where to insert the needle?

Landmarks on the body and measurements using the hand and fingers as a ruler make point location not only a healing art, but a well-defined science. Of course, the ability to locate deeper and more profoundly responsive points *under* the skin requires experience and skill.

Are points found only along Channels?

All twelve Organ channels and two of the Eight Extra channels have their own points. Also, there are numbers of "Miscellaneous" and "New" Points, not associated with these meridians. It is of interest that the remaining six from the Eight "Extra," cross and share Organ channel points.

Can you treat points without needles?

Pressure, heat, ice, laser, ultrasound, and electricity applied to the acupuncture points can be used to cause the desired physiological effects. Needling, however, offers a way to control Qi energy that, while being relatively more invasive, is one which many acupuncturists believe is the most effective.

How many points are there on the body?

Channel points total 365. If you add the Miscellaneous, New Points and micro-acupuncture systems, there are approximately two thousand.

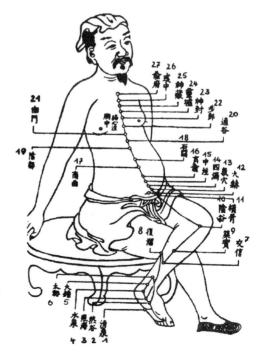

Traditional chart of the Kidney Channel

Essence (Jing), Spirit (Shen) and Fluids

Western medicine explains aging, when not caused by disease, as involving a built-in time clock. What does acupuncture theory say about aging and longevity?

At birth we inherit a supply of Prenatal or Inherited Qi that combines with postnatal Qi energy (the Acquired Qi that comes from food and from the air we breathe) to implement growth and life itself. Known as "Jing" and translated as Essence, this substance is responsible for maturation and the sexual functions. As one gets older, one's Jing becomes weaker. This can be seen in the outward signs of aging. However, certain acupuncture methods and the use of herbs can help to nourish the Essence and prolong life.

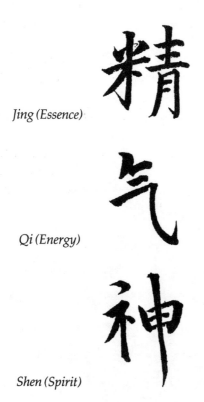

Jing (Essence)

Qi (Energy)

Shen (Spirit)

In Chinese culture, caligraphy is much more than elegant penmanship. It is a fine art as well as an expression of the individual's personality and state of being. The spontaneous gesture of the hand that produces the drawn character expresses the exact state of the caligrapher's Qi-energy.

Will you explain the Chinese concept of Spirit? Is it a religious term?

Spirit (Shen) is the brilliance, vigor and drive behind human expression, in the mind and in the emotions. It means something like our word "spirit" in such uses as "He played the violin with great spirit" or "the soccer team showed great spirit." It serves as a Yang complement to Yin Essence (Jing). Spirit, Essence and Qi are considered to be the family jewels bestowed on us as our natural birthright. Spirit is thus not treated in the context of religious cult, though the word "Shen," as the word "spirit" in English, also can refer to "spiritual" entities.

With the Communist Revolution, Mainland China became a secular culture. For many years the Communist government suppressed organized religions such as the various forms of Taoism and Buddhism. Today there is a greater tolerance of many traditional religious practices by the authorities, and adherents can safely continue their rituals.

The formal practice of these religions, however, must be distinguished, for instance, from Taoist philosophical and cultural values regarding harmonious existence. These have influenced Chinese culture generally and Chinese medicine in particular, apart from religious observances.

Aspects of life that in the West may be considered of a fundamentally religious character, China has treated with scientific scrutiny. Thus the scientific studies of Traditional Chinese Medicine did not shrink from investigations of the "spirit."

What is the significant of the Body Fluids?

Acupuncture uses the general expression "Body Fluids" in reference to all liquids found in a person other than Blood. However, like Blood, Body Fluids are considered to be Yin and dependent upon the Yang of Qi to put them in motion. These substances include perspiration, saliva, digestive juices, urine, and tears. Needed for lubrication and secretion, Body Fluids function with several Tissues and Organs. If the Fluids become too Yang, they lose their liquidity and disorders result such as coughing, dry skin, and constipation. In general, Fluids lubricate, moisten and sustain vicinities of the body that would ordinarily suffer dryness. Dampness/Dryness clinically constitute two diagnostic signs.

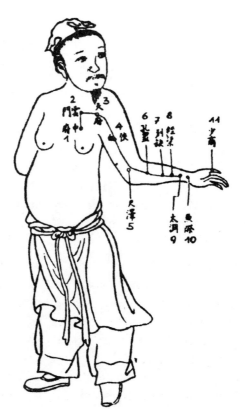

Traditional chart of the Lung Channel

3

Dysfunction of Specific Organs

The Kidney

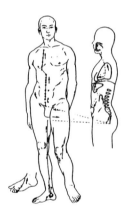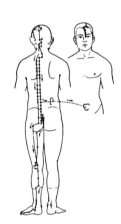

Kidney Channel   *Urinary Bladder Channel*

The Kidney is singled out from among the Organ energy systems because it is the primary source of Qi energy in the body. All the other Organs depend in one way or another on the Kidney.

While acupuncture in general is concerned with the integration of the energies from all the Organs, the Kidney is still special, because everything is affected by Kidney power. It regulates the Heart, takes Qi from the Lung, invigorates the Lung and Spleen, and nourishes the Liver. More than any other Organ, it rules our existence.

In connection with the Kidney, special mention should be made of the concept of sexuality in acupuncture. As in Western medical science, sexuality encompasses reproduction, gender differences, and the gratification of physical desires. But in Chinese thought, the energies involved in sexuality are also concerned with self-development and what we would call personal growth. Sexuality is associated with the Kidney, which includes not only the organs designated in Western medicine by that name, but also the genitals. According to acupuncture, general vitality, sexual energy, reproduction, and the potentiality for self-development all dwell in the Essence or Jing of a person, which is a special, life-giving substance that the Kidney stores. Therefore, the Kidney takes charge of sexuality, reproduction, vitality, and personal growth. Jing flows abundantly in youth and declines in old age. The Kidney as a storehouse of Jing is considered a Yin function. Kidney Organ Qi, in Yang fashion, activates Jing. The Kidney's role is to direct this action.

Can acupuncture deal with infertility?

"I am a married woman in my 30's, trying to conceive without much success. The local fertility clinic tells me that I should have the physical ability to give birth, with the help of hormone supplements. My husband's sperm was tested as normal. Now, after five years of no birth control, nothing has happened. If relevant, for years I have experienced irregular menstruation. My medical history also shows emotional depression and chills even in hot weather."

An entire subdivision of acupuncture provides care in gynecology and obstetrics. In Chinese medicine, your menstrual problem would definitely be considered to be connected to your infertility. For conception to take place, the womb needs sufficient Blood and Qi energy. Your chills suggest poor circulation in general. In addition, your troubled emotions very likely stagnate Liver Qi.

Acupuncture in fact can help both the physical body and the emotions. The regulation of your monthly cycle and the activation of Blood flow by acupuncture combined with nourishing herbs should produce results.

Speaking in terms of Organs, infertility commonly stems from the Liver, Spleen and Kidney. The Liver stores Blood, the Spleen manufactures Blood, and the Kidney oversees the whole process of reproduction. Two non-Organ, "Extra" channels work closely with menstruation and infertility. One of these, "the Conception Vessel," manages conception as its name suggests, but requires Blood and Qi. The other is the "Penetrating Vessel." This takes Blood from the Liver to form a reservoir that supplies the Conception Vessel.

Can acupuncture help male sexual problems?

"I'm a young guy in my early twenties with a lot of financial obliga-tions for my family. The fear of losing my job worries me constantly. It's also depressing that I cannot find a better job to make more money. Anyhow, my personal problem is in the bedroom. It seems that I just can't keep an erection for good sex. Sometimes I can't even get it up. In spite of this, I'm healthy, physically strong and athletic, but certain nights I feel a little dizzy, sleepless and nauseous. Can you help me?"

Any degree of impotence comes from a lack of energy associ-ated with the Kidney. The anxiety which has entered your mind takes its toll and harms the Kidney. Possibly Liver, Spleen and Heart weaknesses have followed. These Organs carry importance for sexual functions, since they influence Blood circulation. Diffi-culties with them is shown by the symptoms of depression, dizzi-ness, worry, nausea and insomnia.

By restoring normal Kidney Qi, acupuncture has proven effec-tive in correcting impotence. Acupuncturists frequently stimulate a point in the lower abdomen, which brings forth the Inherited Qi energy to assist performance. We would also recommend treatment to motivate the Liver and other deficiencies to improve the flow of Blood. In your case, we would strengthen the emotions too.

Can a pregnant woman receive acupuncture needles?

Acupuncture helps pregnancy related ailments, from morning sickness to prolonged labor and difficult delivery. Certain acupuncture points, however, should not be used during the entire pregnancy, and others should be avoided during specific months.

Can acupuncture alleviate the discomforts of menopause?

Chinese medicine makes adjustments relating to the "biological clock" in women—the long term processes of growth and aging—by managing two special channels with Kidney energy. The channels are the "Penetrating" and "Conception" Vessels. At different phases of life, changes happen to the Penetrating Vessel's supply of Blood and the Conception Vessel's support of fertility. In a young girl, Kidney Qi blossoms. This leads the way for the Conception Vessel to receive Blood from the Penetrating Vessel. When this occurs (at the preteen or early teen years), monthly periods start. When old-age depletes Kidney Qi, there is a decline in menstruation.

Kidney Qi divides into Cold Yin and Hot Yang. A decline in one aspect will expand the other. With menopausal symptoms such as hot flashes and lower back pain, the Yin has declined, overloading the body with Yang. Consequently, hot and dry symptoms appear such as afternoon fever and dry skin. Since the Kidney sits in the low back, pain occurs here and may also be felt in the knees. Also, Kidney Qi "opens" to the ears causing the ringing in the ears Western medicine knows as "tinnitus."

After a thorough evaluation, acupuncture will nourish the Kidney Yin for fluid lubrication and coolness. Then adjustments to the Penetrating and Conception Vessels will help eliminate symptoms.

The Liver

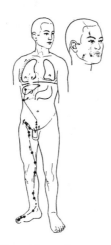 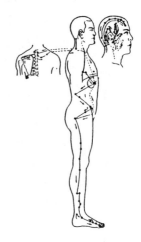

Liver Channel *Gall Bladder Channel*

Can acupuncture help menstrual problems?

"As an active woman with irregular and painful menstrual periods, I have an additional problem of a constantly bloated abdomen. I feel discomfort in this area and below the rib cage. My hot temper seems to aggravate the pain. I think that in some way my emotions affect the swelling. Can this be true?"

Your emotions definitely act to mold your disorder. Thousands of years ago, Chinese medicine grew aware of the body-mind connection.

From the symptoms you mention, I see a Liver problem — not in regard to the structure or chemistry of the Organ, but with its energy. The Liver works to spread Qi and Blood. Self-induced angry negative feelings interrupt this healthy circulation. When your Organ's energy suffers a traffic jam, accumulations pile up and stick out as lumps or masses. Because the Liver stores Blood, stagnation also will interfere with the menstrual flow.

Acupuncture arouses Liver stagnancy and gets things moving again. It can also calm your anger. Your distended abdomen, menstrual problems, and pain should subside after a series of visits.

Can acupuncture cure migraines?

"For a few years I've been having terrible migraine headaches. I get dizzy at times and recently noticed some blurry vision and ringing in my ears. My doctor treats me for hypertension and nervousness, and my eyes are checked periodically. Funny sensations happen to me late in the day. My hands and feet feel warm and I experience a slight fever. I would really like to be cured of my annoying complaints."

Your symptoms result from a Liver imbalance. The Organ's cool Yin has diminished, inflating the Ascending Liver Yang. You are suffering from *overactive* and *hot* Yang. Liver energy rises. Going to the head internally, this rising force leaves you with migraine and vision problems. Fever also relates to too much Yang.

Liver energy opens to the eyes, but the Gallbladder Channel (the channel of the Organ that complements the Liver) surrounds the ear. Ringing in the ear can occur from channel disharmony. Also, the Kidney opens in the ear. In the Cycle of the Organs known as the "Nourishing Cycle," the Kidney precedes the Liver. At times, reduced Kidney Yin lowers Liver Yin—a shared imbalance between two Organs.

Nourishing the Yin and cooling down the Yang regulates the body. Acupuncture needling may treat both the Liver and Kidney as well as the Gallbladder. If untreated, or treated without success, I'm sorry to say the imbalances could lead to serious conditions in the form of stroke and coma.

How does acupuncture deal with stroke?

"My grandfather had a stroke which left him without the use of an arm. His speech became slurry and he has a slight paralysis of the face. I always knew him as a strong and forceful man, who only got treated for high blood pressure. Can acupuncture help? He was in a coma for awhile and has received physical therapy for rehabilitation."

Conventional Western medicine interprets a stroke as a clot in a blood vessel of the brain, or as cerebral bleeding. Chinese medicine understands the basis of a stroke as an Organ mishap. Like a volcano, Liver Yang shoots up and produces two internal damages. First, the heat of Yang congeals Fluids to form Phlegm. Second, Yang turns into Wind. Together, Wind and Phlegm block the flow of Qi and Blood, which disables the patient. The generation of internal Wind is such an important factor that acupuncture names the disease "central wind."

Immediately after a stroke, First-aid needling can open Channels and soothe the stirring of Wind. Whether during the crisis situation or in follow-up care, acupuncture reduces Wind upheaval through Liver control and restores the current of normalized Qi and Blood. We also solicit aid from the Spleen to dry obstacles relating to Phlegm.

Rehabilitation through acupuncture will address each symptom. To energize your grandfather's arm, needling specific points irrigates Qi and Blood. Scalp acupuncture techniques recently have been shown to be effective in treating stroke. Since the Heart extends to the tongue, Heart Qi assists the return of speech. An acupuncturist's awareness of related energy systems will help in many ways.

How does acupuncture deal with gallstones?

As Yin-Yang partners, the Liver and Gallbladder interact with one another and participate in the formation of gallstones. The Gallbladder stores bile, and Damp Heat can settle where it's not wanted. In the presence of Damp Heat, bile hardens with painful symptoms. Initial causes originate from the associated emotion of anger and the Liver's loss of its ability to scatter Qi. Stagnant Stomach Qi and a greasy diet can bring about the disorder also.

Correction consists of Damp Heat drainage and Liver Qi stimulation. For decades Western surgery has removed gallstones, but records reveal a large percentage of recurrence. Upon the deletion of Damp Heat and the restoration of the Liver's ability to disperse energy, a cure should remain permanent.

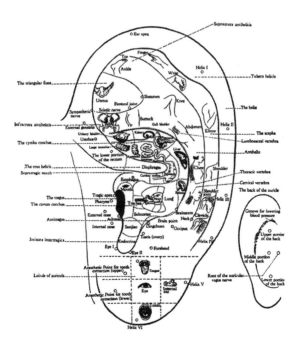

Acupuncture points on the ear. Oriental Medicine employs several specialized subsystems of acupuncture points. Each of these accesses the energy of the whole body through specific, external bodily parts such as the hand, the foot, and the ear.

Can acupuncture deal with seizures?

"At an early age, my child had seizures with jerking movements of his arms and legs. I was relieved to be told that he had no problems of the nervous system such as meningitis. Instead, hypocalcemia was found, for which he took calcium. Now at three years old he still shakes. What can be done?"

For seizures right after birth, doctors consider infections or defects in the development of the brain and spinal cord likely. Other causes are found to be metabolic problems involving minerals that can affect nerves as in this case of hypocalcemia. Hypocalcemia means a lack of calcium in the blood. Parathyroid glands (glands at the sides of the thyroid) regulate calcium.

The medical evaluation of your son's condition was based on the anatomy of nerves and the chemistry of endocrine glands, but not on a direct consideration of the symptom, the shaking itself. Chinese medicine understands such conditions as indicating the presence of "Wind" in the channels. As breezes make leaves flutter, internal Wind stirs seizures.

By the specific characteristics of the symptoms, acupuncturists detect the internal sources generating the Wind and the drafts through afflicted channels. Often disorders of this kind relate to the Liver and to energy passages along the spine. The problem will subside following Wind removal and channel adjustments. Normalizing the internal environment will also result in the presence of more calcium showing up in the lab tests.

The Heart

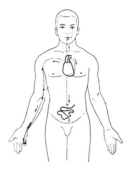

Heart Channel

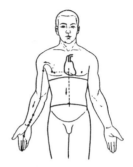

Pericardium Channel

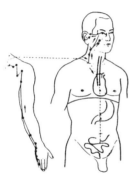

Small Intestine Channel

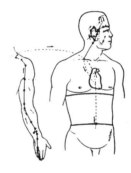

Tripple Heater Channel

How does the Western understanding of the causes and treatment of heart disease compare with that of acupuncture?

American medicine keeps the ailing heart pumping with aerobic exercise, low-fat diet, and by-pass surgery, not to mention pacemakers. Recent medical research sheds new light on how emotional stress disturbs the heart.

According to China's ancient understanding, the Heart is far more than a Blood pump and the focus of emotional stress. The Heart houses the Spirit of life. It holds the reigns of the mind and the talking tongue. It is the control center for all of our emotions. It invigorates and rules the functions of Blood circulation, the Blood vessels, and the Spirit.

How does acupuncture treat hardening of the coronary arteries and its symptoms: feeling cold, shortness of breath, tiredness? I am being treated with a vasodilator.

Coronary arteries provide circulation and oxygen for the heart muscle. They serve as the heart's own vascular system. When these vessels harden in the condition known as arteriosclerosis, the artery may narrow or create a blockage.

There's much conjecture in Western medicine as to the cause. Acupuncture's understanding of the balancing and passing of energy gives us further insight. In arteriosclerosis, the Heart's invigorating Yang energy has dropped and shifted to a mode of laid-back Yin Qi.

According to acupuncture, the Kidney regulates the Heart. A common observation by Western doctors shows that kidney failure often follows cardiac insufficiency. Western medicine cannot explain this connection.

Acupuncture treats Heart problems by restoring active Yang, which should reduce the symptoms. In strengthening Kidney Yang, the Heart Yang will take the needed power from its supplier.

Can acupuncture treat sleeplessness?

"At night I toss and turn and cannot fall asleep. Fatigue sets in during the day. Friends tell me I look washed-out. I have tried sleeping pills, which relax me but clearly have not really changed anything. And when I sleep, I often wake up with nightmares. What's wrong?"

Your insomnia and exhausted, pale appearance point to deficient Heart Blood. The Spirit sheltered in your Heart must receive more Blood. Then a nourished Spirit will allow a peaceful rest. Basically, acupuncture can needle areas to revive adequate circulation in the chest, which we call the Upper Warmer. Supplemental points may include the use of specific herbs for insomnia and a method to *equalize* Yin energy at night and Yang during the day.

Can acupuncture treat urinary tract infections accompanied by high fever?

"My problem is a recurrent urinary tract infection, sometimes with high fever. The heat I sense can be blazing. A degree of relief comes with antibiotics, but the condition returns without warning. Besides seeing a urologist, I'm in psychotherapy. I'm sure that Chinese medicine would categorize my neurosis in the Heart and Fire Element. Right?"

True, but both your ailments belong in that Element. It's Fire with Fire. The Heart and Small Intestine share a Yin-Yang relationship. Small Intestine energy separates the pure from the impure. This process makes urine for deposit in the Urinary Bladder. Since Fire can drop into the Organ, symptoms of infection result with Damp Heat. So heat in the Heart causes psychological disorders, and in the Small Intestine, urinary infections.

An acupuncturist will drain the excess Fire and regulate your Organ-Element Cycle. The Kidney and Urinary Bladder in the Water Element probably are due for a tune-up.

Spleen and Stomach

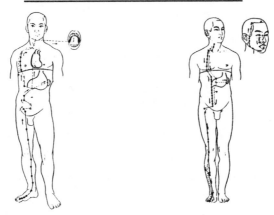

Spleen Channel   Stomach Channel

How does acupuncture treat stomach ulcers?

"My husband and I work in executive positions and share the same stress-related ailment. We have both been diagnosed with a stomach ulcer. What I do not understand are the gross differences between us as we try to accommodate this nuisance. I feel better when eating warm food and drinking hot coffee or tea. Pressure and warmth to the outside of my stomach relieves pain and I crave warmer weather. My husband, who incidentally is diabetic, moves in the opposite direction. He likes to drink cold beverages and prefers a cooler environment. Any explanations or advice?"

A Western medical diagnosis, based mainly on structural and chemical findings, with some awareness of the stress factor is helpful up to a point: it aids in locating symptoms for acupuncture treatment. But comprehending the body's internal environment presents a clearer picture. Your disorder very likely arises from Cold or decreased Yang in the Spleen and Stomach. In your husband's case, Heat or Fire within the Stomach motivates his drive for coolness. Heat also dries Fluids as part of the disease process of diabetes. Either of these separate states of internal atmosphere can ulcerate the stomach lining. Further questioning with pulse and tongue examinations would yield a more exact evaluation.

You may find permanent help from acupuncture and Chinese dietary suggestions. Meanwhile, your individual choices for food, drink, and surroundings actually seem to be following Chinese medical principles, which temporarily regulate the cold-hot imbalance. Apart from the emotional factor, in regard to your case, cold sources of a gastric ulcer often stem from excessive raw food and harmful seasonal invasions. In your husband's case, alcohol and rich delicacies may be igniting Fire. By warming a cold body or cooling down the heat, some relief results.

Everything in me seems to droop down: my abdomen is sinking, I have hemorrhoids and what my doctor calls a prolapse uterus. Also I bleed easily. What can acupuncture do for me?

The Spleen corresponds to the element Earth. As the earth supports everything upon the planet, the Spleen provides Organs and Blood *ground* to stand on. When parts of the body fall out of position, we consider this to be due to shortages of the Qi of the Spleen. This force holds Organs in their place and Blood in its Vessel. Your Spleen obviously needs strengthening. Acupuncture will adjust the Organ and lift up the downward shift in energy.

What causes retention of fluid, according to acupuncture?

"My arms and legs swell with water. I cough excessively to clear my throat of mucus. After years of taking diuretic pills, I still carry a lot of fluid."

You have an underactive Spleen. Among the Spleen's normal actions is a drying potency. In effect, moisture disturbs the Spleen, but, in contrast, it gets a big welcome from the Stomach. One needs dryness, the other needs wetness. Corrections to the Spleen and Stomach, plus work with the indicated diuretic points, in all likelihood will eliminate the surplus of water.

How does acupuncture treat constipation and diarrhea?

"I vacillate between constipation and diarrhea and often feel a kind of tummy ache. When I apply pressure there, it's better for awhile. I suffer from fatigue and often have chills. My doctor says I have an intestinal virus."

An evaluation by an acupuncturist will show weak energy of the Large Intestine. Transferring Qi to the depleted Organ ought to relieve your ailments. It sounds as if you need a shot of energy in general.

Can acupuncture help relieve diabetic symptoms like constant thirst, hunger, and frequent urination?

For centuries, acupuncture has corrected the symptoms you mention and has restored normal functions to the Pancreas. One reason why China did not completely accept Western medicine had to do with the West's lack of methods for rehabilitating the damage caused by *degenerative* diseases such as diabetes. Medical minds in the West think directly in terms of chemistry and artificial replacements. Thus, insulin from out-of-body sources substitutes for what the body cannot produce naturally.

Acupuncturists recognize in diabetes failing Yin Organs with too much Yang heat. Also well-known is the association of the Triple Warmer with these specific symptoms. In diabetes, heat dries up certain Organ Fluids that include insulin—it is like a drought that evaporates a slowly moving river.

The basic disturbance revolves around the Kidney. Yin and Qi deficiencies here result in the excess passage of urine and diabetic related symptoms of back pain, blurred vision, fatigue and a weak speaking voice. Heat in the Spleen-Stomach area causes hunger. Heat in the Lung causes thirst. Traditional Chinese physicians termed the diabetic condition, "thirsting and wasting disease."

An internally arid and disturbed environment being the cause, you may ask, what causes the cause? The answer is found partly in diet and partly in emotion. Large amounts of fatty and rich foods and alcohol interfere with the transportation functions of digestion. Food particles pile up and turn to Heat. To dwell on harmful emotions will stagnate Qi energy; harmful emotions and stagnate Qi both produce Fire. Added injury occurs from physical exhaustion at work and at sexual pursuits.

Western medicine has recorded diabetic tendencies in families. These may show conditioned eating and work habits, emotional patterns, and responses with inherited weaknesses.

Acupuncture treats diabetes by cooling down the Fire and rehabilitating Organ Yin. The Spleen often is referred to as the "Spleen-Pancreas," since their activities are connected. Treating precise Pancreas acupuncture points proves helpful together with herbs that moisten Yin and nourish Organ Fluids.

The Lung

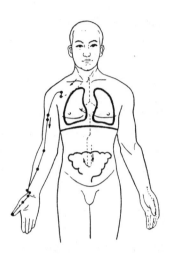

Lung Channel

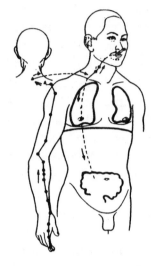

Large Intestine Channel

Can acupuncture cure the common cold?

> *"The cure for the common cold has eluded generations of medical researchers. Medications to kill the cold virus are sought, but nothing comes forward except antihistamines, vitamin C and cough drops. If the cold turns to pneumonia or bronchitis, we take antibiotics. But people die from pneumonia, caught even after being admitted to a hospital. Antibiotics have their limitations. How does acupuncture handle these respiratory diseases?"*

Western medicine looks at structure and microbes and labels a disorder according to the afflicted anatomy and the afflicting agent. It calls inflammation to the larynx "laryngitis," to the bronchial tubes "bronchitis," to the lungs, "pneumonia" ("pneumon" means lung) and so on. Viruses or bacteria add to the name, so we get "viral pneumonia." But the common cold is not located precisely and may have several causes.

Chinese medicine assesses the environment and Organ Qi. Illnesses of respiration involve the Lung in those two ways, outwardly and inwardly. Outwardly, there are the direct invasions of Cold, Heat, Wind and Damp, and the combinations thereof. Depending on what type of harm enters our Lungs, certain symptoms appear in response. For example, Cold that annoys the Lung will produce chills and a runny nose. Heat will result in a high fever, a sore, dry throat, and congested nasal mucus. Inwardly and more seriously are flaws in the Lung Organ itself that result in asthma, tuberculosis and emphysema. Whether caused externally or internally, any disorder of respiration develops from lowered immunity.

Therapy, which may apply herbs, moxa heat, and cupping, together with acupuncture needling, pulls out the destructive atmosphere and builds up Lung Qi. Since the Kidney grabs inhalation energy from the Lung and roots the breath, we often tone up the Kidney too. Another source of aid to dry Phlegm comes from the Spleen.

A protective Qi surrounds the body. The Lung, with its complement, the Large Intestine, controls this outer energy shield. Points along their Channels thus affect the immune system.

Some speculation here may provide an answer as to why patients get pneumonia once they're in the hospital. Pneumonia is frequent especially among the elderly. Western medicine explains this by cross-contamination between patients or stagnation in the chest from lack of exercise. Acupuncture notices daily Blood withdrawal from an area of the inner arm that corresponds to the sedation point of the Lung. Although routine blood tests present information used by the doctor, repeatedly using this place for vein puncture may weaken the Lung and allow pneumonia.

Can acupuncture treat allergies that affect the respiratory system?

Acupuncture can be of help. Allergies in general relate to the Lungs. Allergic respiratory problems center on deficient Lung energy, which opens to the nose and governs the voice.

Can acupuncture treat skin disorders?

"A lingering skin disorder on my elbows and knees has a diagnosis of psoriasis, also eczema or dermatitis. The normally prescribed treatment consists of strong cortisone cream with an occasional antihistamine taken by mouth. Sometimes it appears cured, but too often it flares up terribly. Is there something else that can be done?"

According to Chinese medicine, skin problems unfold because of toxins retained within us. Organs largely responsible for their elimination are the Lung and Large Intestine. When wastes cannot leave by regular means, they surface through the skin. Therefore, acupuncturists stimulate these Organs of excretion. Enhancement of Blood circulation and protective Qi adds to the correction.

Acupuncture assigns the Lung and Large Intestine to the Element, Metal. For practical purposes, miners dig out the earth's metal. With similar actions, the Lung and Large Intestine extract toxins and waste from the body.

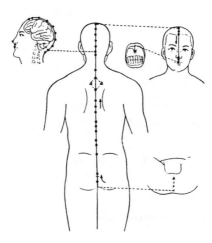

Du Channel

Can acupuncture treat emotions like grief and sadness?

"People say I'm a workaholic. After hours, I fit aerobic exercise into my schedule, and there's still time for more sports, theater and concerts. My predominant emotion is sadness as a result of a lot of tragedy in my life. When I'm not occupied with something, the grief gets out of hand. What really bothers me, though, is that I wake up almost every morning exactly at 3:00 A. M. What's happening?"

Each Organ in Chinese medicine interconnects with an emotion. Sadness belongs to the Lung.

To understand why you awake at three in the morning, we must know how energy flows. The Cycle of Organ Elements *(see page 50)* shows how the control and movement of the Qi occurs in accordance with the laws of nature's five progressive phases. Energy also circulates through the channels according to the time of day. Organ meridians prevail alternately for two hour segments.

The twenty-four hour cycle begins at 3:00 A.M. with the Lung. Your Lung Qi undoubtedly overacts when its time period arrives. Adjustments to fix the imbalance and regulate your emotional disturbance are possible with acupuncture. The measures of bi-hourly times for all Organ meridians are listed in the table on pages 52-53.

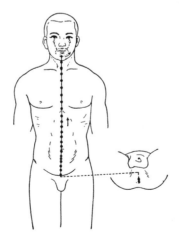

Ren Channel

The Glands

A group of glands releases secretions called hormones into the circulating blood. They are the *endocrine* glands, and they work together as the *endocrine* system. Among these we have the pituitary, thyroid, parathyroid and adrenal glands, and the gonads for egg and sperm development. Found in the head, neck, abdomen, and sexual organs, the endocrine glands secrete hormones that regulate growth, sex, reproduction and metabolism.

Interesting theories have recently been advanced claiming that acupuncture acts fundamentally on the endocrine system. Chinese medical practice, it is alleged, really works through glandular reactions. As with similar attempts to understand acupuncture in terms of the nervous system, we must remember that Western medical theory stops at structure and chemistry and does not address the whole world of Qi energy. The endocrine system is certainly profoundly affected by acupuncture techniques. But it is Qi energy that is responsible for these affects. Here is the acupuncture-glandular connection: energy influences internal secretions.

Certain Organs maintain particularly close relations with certain glands, as is the case for instance with the Spleen and Pancreas. Another Organ that works very closely with the glands is the Triple Warmer. Since energy adjusts imbalances in each of the Three Warmers, we can correlate activities of Triple Warmer Qi with those of the glands. To know the functions of these "Burners" well is to know much about acupuncture physiology. The Upper Burner manages respiration through the Heart and Lungs. The Spleen and Stomach in the Middle Burner control digestion. Down in the Lower Burner, the Kidney and Liver occupy functions of reproduction and elimination.

The adrenal gland sits on top of the kidney, so won't the Kidney affect the adrenal?

Yes; however, the impact of Organ Qi travels far and wide and is not limited to the proximity of the Organ. To understand this, let's compare the Western concept of the "master gland" to the Chinese concept of "master Organ." Early biochemistry and physiology honored the pituitary with the title "master gland," because its hormones act strongly on other glands. In more recent times, research has shown the hypothalamus to be the true "leader," who even "rules" the pituitary.

In the Chinese system, as "master Organ," the Kidney directs all glands including the hypothalamus, pituitary and adrenal. In fact, the Kidney and its related Channels energize the entire endocrine system. Consequently, Kidney deficiencies will impair any gland's power as, for instance, in hypopituitarism, where short supplies from the pituitary stunt physical growth and sexual development. Other "hypo-" (deficient) conditions also can be traced to declined Kidney Qi.

Can acupuncture explain why the adrenal glands secrete two substances with opposite effects—cortisone and adrenaline?

They can indeed. Yin-Yang characterizes visible matter as well as invisible forces. The adrenal gland is divided in two *structural* parts. Each part secretes a different hormone; one is Yin the other Yang. Cortisone from the cortex is the Yin hormone and it calms down flared-up inflammation. In-office injections of synthetic cortisone creates the same anti-inflammatory process. Adrenaline is the Yang hormone, produced in the adrenal gland's medulla.

If you need a natural shot of Yang, call on the adrenal's medulla. Adrenaline (incidentally, the first isolated hormone, and the first one artificially made) speeds up the heart and raises blood pressure.

How does Qi act to stimulate the adrenal gland?

"I know that Cushing's disease results from too much cortisone and Addison's disease, which afflicted the late President John F. Kennedy, from too little. I know the chemistry, but what about the invisible forces of Qi that act upon the adrenal gland and its cortex?"

As for *invisible forces*, consider the prefixes "hypo" and "hyper" that appear on several names of endocrine disorders. "Hypo" means too little; "hyper" means too much. These prefixes correspond to the acupuncture concepts of excess and dificiency, specifically of Yin or Yang Organ energy. Deficient Kidney Yang hampers normal fiery actions and causes the hyper- (increased) release of cold, fluid Yin. When Kidney Yin takes a plunge, empty Yang emerges producing overactive evaporation and hypo- (decreased) moisture.

Insight into the Yin-Yang "pulley" tells us why glandular problems happen. Too much secretion of cortisone from the adrenal cortex (Yang down, Yin up) forms excess disorders to bring about Cushing's disease. Sufferers display a frail skin and a pale, rounded face. The opposite condition—the underactive production of this hormone—gives rise to Addison's disease. The signs of Addison's disease—a certain skin pigmentation, weight loss and dehydration—reflect lowered Yin and an inflation of hot-drying Yang.

Treatments concentrate on a special area of life force, which embodies Qi from our ancestors. Kidney administration supervises this inherited Qi. It is stored by the Kidney and partly resides in the Eight Extra Channels. Adjustments in some of these Vessels and on the Kidney Organ itself, provide desired therapy for glandular problems.

Can acupuncture deal with thyroid problems?

"My blood pressure is high and I do not sleep well. Warm sensations and sweating at night make me irritable. A medical opinion has suggested surgical removal of the thyroid, although there is no sign of a tumor. I thought an enlarged thyroid could be controlled with iodine supplements. Can acupuncture help? Should I undergo the surgery?"

As a science of the physical body and its chemistry, in considering thyroid disorders Western medicine looks for excesses and decreases of hormone production and metabolism. Examinations may also probe the essential tissues of the gland. Located in the neck, the thyroid controls the rate of metabolism in all your cells. The thyroid demands iodine to make its major hormone called thyroxine. Current therapy for an enlarged thyroid prescribes anti-thyroid drugs and iodine. Treatments may incorporate thyroid hormone replacements.

Both hyperthyroidism (over-active thyroid) also called "goiter" and Grave's disease, and hypothyroidism (under-active thyroid) also called myxedema, can distend (enlarge) the gland. Iodine treats both conditions perfectly well. Acupuncture, however, goes beyond correcting glandular chemistry and structure and assesses the total internal environment. Both Chinese and Western medicine see connections between emotional upset and hyperthyroidism. However, Chinese medicine is more precise in that it understands how specific emotional problems are connected to the energy of specific Organs. Psychological stress causes the flow of Liver Qi to stagnate in the Channels. This stagnation then changes to Fire.

From your description, I would say your symptoms show a definite Heart energy disruption. Stagnant Fire shrivels Heart Yin, which, in turn, expands Heart Yang Fire. Hypertension (high blood pressure), insomnia, feverish feelings, night sweats and irritability indicate this pattern. In the sequence of the disease process, Liver Qi stagnates and converts to a general Fire that injures Heart Yin and causes a complication of Heart Fire. Meanwhile, the general Fire causes Phlegm to gather and Blood to stagnate. Goiter appears when Phlegm and Blood clog Channels of the neck.

Acupuncture treatment would drain all the Fires, clear Phlegm and stagnation, rehabilitate the fallen Heart Yin, and spread Liver Qi. It may sound strange to Western ears, but that's how acupuncture works. Your symptoms should subside after a series of treatments. They should not require surgery.

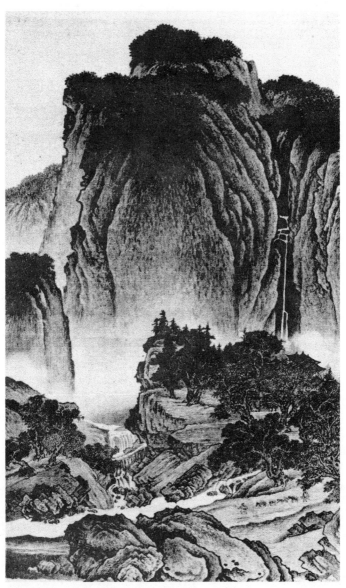

Wang Shih-min, after Fan K'uan's Travelers among Streams and Mountains. *(Undated, late 1620s)*

4

Children and Acupuncture

Do you find that children accept acupuncture?

Some of my greatest satisfactions in practice come from patient feedback. It is especially true when youngsters tell me how much better they feel and how they look forward to the acupuncture visits. At times, children accept acupuncture more willingly than grownups. Their energy flows with the vitality of new life. With innocent sensitivity, they feel themselves go through a healing process. Without the association of needles with pain found in conditioned Western adult populations, many infants, toddlers and young children love to be helped by acupuncture.

Is acupuncture administered differently to adults and children?

Certainly. Children are susceptible to different illnesses than adults. Disorders such as tonsillitis, whooping cough, obstructed digestion, mumps, measles, bed-wetting and hyperactivity dominate a list of childhood diseases. During adulthood, a different set of problems surface. Since changes in energy and Organ function carry the responsibility for these changes in illness, there are corresponding variations in treatment.

When ailments are similar between young and mature patients, the selection of acupuncture points to be needled is likely to be similar too. In general, children respond with fewer stimulations and within a shorter period of time. Of major consideration is the fact that, with children, emotionally related causes for illness have not had an opportunity to harden. An adult, for instance, may need help dealing with deep-seated bitterness and its physical consequences. In contrast, therapy for the young deals more with problems of Organ Qi development, and growth of the body, mind and spirit. It also frequently deals with the high fever of diseases associated with the excessive Yang of youth.

Can acupuncture be used on babies?

Acupuncture knows no age limit. Infants often respond well, since the first bursts of life's energy respond well to the acupuncturist's direction.

What basic differences are there between American and Chinese approaches to pediatrics?

American medicine, child care included, largely works with visible structure. When children get sick, diagnoses tend to be given in terms of viruses, bacteria, problems with body chemistry and body tissue. Common forms of therapy make use of antibiotics, pills for pain and fever, casts to immobilize injuries, surgery and psychotherapy.

Chinese medicine, child care included, pays attention to the balance of Yin and Yang, Organ energy, and internal environmental qualities such as hot, cold, dry and damp.

Symptoms are looked at in terms of the patterns into which they fit. Upon evaluation, acupuncture regulates disharmonies and strengthens Organs. Although Western pediatrics and acupuncture record the same symptoms, the way they define diseases and choose treatments are poles apart.

What are the differences in the ways Western medicine and acupuncture categorize childhood diseases?

Acupuncture applies a totally different set of categories to the symptoms in small children than Western medicine does and therefore arrives at different connections between them. (This is of course true of the acupuncture in relation to adults as well.) For instance, one important category in acupuncture for small children is excess of postnatal Yang. We see it in high fevers, inflammatory conditions, and hyperactive behavior. Overabundant Yang produces abnormal heat, which may turn to emotional excitement and/or to a rise in body temperature. If excess Yang bothers children emotionally, they exhibit agitation, anxiety, crying at night, nightmares, fear of the dark and sleeplessness. Associated Kidney and Heart disharmonies usually uncover psychological sources. Too much Yang in body parts causes convulsions, mumps, nose bleed, meningitis, chicken pox and various feverish diseases. Of course, Yang combined with Damp allows the breeding of infections recognized by Western medicine. All these problems are seen in acupuncture as due ultimately to excess postnatal Yang, whereas

Western medicine would see no particular connection between infectious diseases, for instance, and behavioral or psychological problems.

Other contributors to the pains of growing that in Western medicine are considered congenital deformities are viewed similarly in acupuncture, except that the congenital factor in acupuncture is Inherited Qi. In Western medicine, faulty organs are often thought to be responsible for illnesses pertaining to digestion, respiration and urination. But in acupuncture, allergies may also be on this list since they, for example, may come from ailing Lungs.

As in Western medicine, acupuncturists look for harmful invasions, poor diets, stress and congenital or inherited handicaps. Also, in acupuncture, deficiencies at birth generally mean deficiency in Inherited Qi. Weaknesses in Organ function and the flow of energy can result from a variety of individual deficiencies in the parents. Before birth, prenatal sustenance depends on the umbilical cord and the passing of ancestral energy to the unborn child. If this energy is damaged, it will have its effect in the form of weaknesses in the child. Such weaknesses may not necessarily manifest during infancy. Difficulties may arise later on as asthma, skeletal defects, neuromuscular disabilities, juvenile diabetes and mental retardation.

Can acupuncture, applied to the mother before the birth of her child, help the child?

Yes. Before birth, acupuncture has a valuable application. Because the mother transfers vital forces to the fetus, acupuncture can strengthen this process. Needling a certain point at the third and sixth month improves the child's constitutional inheritance. Acupuncturists also avoid certain "forbidden-during-pregnancy" points to prevent damage to fetal energy.

Can acupuncture treat birth defects?

Yes, the body stores Inherited Qi, which remains available throughout life. Acupuncture therapy activates the reserve of forces while it takes help from the Acquired Qi. Certain corrections are possible with this method.

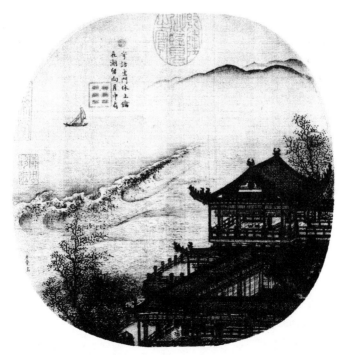

Attributed to Li Sung, The Hangchow Bore in Moonlight.
(Ca. 1210)

What is the acupuncture view on infant immunization by vaccination?

Immunization by vaccination injects a bit of the disease substance to create immunity against that same illness. Often children react by having a moderate case of the affliction. Historically, Chinese medicine discovered a method to prevent small pox before Western science. Still, Chinese medical attitudes show concern for unnecessary risks, but modern practitioners do recognize the actual need for certain inoculations.

If acupuncture has a way to treat a problem successfully and there are no serious threats of permanent damage from the disease, immunization against that problem remains optional. Of course, acupuncture must be available. Measles, mumps, chicken pox and whooping cough are some of the diseases that respond to acupuncture needling. Yet due to the peril of polio paralysis, your child should receive the polio vaccine. This, however, can be taken by mouth.

Chinese medicine opposes the vaccination to prevent measles, for reasons of child development. There are many toxins from pregnancy that stay in the body during the first years after delivery. Measles serves as a release of these harmful accumulations. When there are no brain-damaging complications, acupuncture controls the symptoms of measles very well. The fact that retained poisons could set off future illnesses poses a hazard and should be a matter of thought for parents when deciding on whether or not to inoculate against measles.

Mumps, unlike measles, does not discharge the buildup of toxins. Instead, a gathering of Wind, Damp and Heat settles around the jaw and swells the parotid gland. This is a salivary gland near the ear. Inoculation against mumps, therefore, has gained more acceptance from acupuncturists.

In general, where Chinese medicine treats Organ Qi and internal atmospheric disharmonies, Western medicine goes after the virus. For the well-being of our children, a practical integration of services makes a lot of sense. Competent application of both kinds of health care is the best way to insure the health of a new generation.

Can acupuncture treat bed-wetting?

"My four year-old son has been a bed wetter now for over a year. We've had counseling and visits to specialists, but nothing has helped. Can acupuncture offer an answer?"

Acupuncture treatments can often stop bed-wetting. Some children respond immediately and others need several visits. The evaluation locates inadequate energy in specific Organs. A bad internal environment and negative emotions are often a part of this nightly nuisance.

Organ weakness usually focuses on the Kidney, which controls the Urinary Bladder. Decreases in Kidney Qi and a disappearing warm Kidney Yang permit too much Cold and an inability to hold water. The Lung and Spleen may play a part, since their Qi influences water functions. Damp Heat can disrupt the urinary system. Western medicine would recognize this as a urinary tract infection.

After the exact reason for bed-wetting becomes apparent, the acupuncturist works with the most promising combination of acupuncture points. Needles and moxibustion boost Kidney Yang and push out the unfavorable Cold. Point stimulation regulates the mechanism of the Lung and Spleen to normalize Body Fluids.

Acupuncture also cares for the emotional sensitivities that underlie the problem. Irritability or stress contribute a great deal.

What does Chinese medicine say about hyperactive children?

"My five year-old son is hyperactive and drives me nuts. He cannot sit still, goes wild when he's with other children, and does not do well in school. We tried sedative pills and less sugar and milk in his diet. Our doctor advised us on this, which calmed him down a little."

In Chinese medical terminology, hyperactivity stems from Heat collected in the Heart. The Heart houses the Spirit and mind. The excess Heat causes a high-spirited youngster. At times, Phlegm aggravates this condition. Since sweets and dairy products develop Phlegm, your doctor gave good advice--the less milk and sugar, the less Phlegm for antagonizing effects with Heart Fire. Two other Organs may also be part of the trouble. A poorly working Spleen in a growing child stagnates food and Damp and fires up the Heart. Also, internal Wind from Liver imbalances can stir movements in many directions.

A thorough acupuncture evaluation gets to the core of the problem. Therapy attempts to drain the Heat and calm the Spirit.

How does acupuncture treat tonsillitis and appendicitis?

"Two common surgeries for youngsters are tonsillectomies and appendectomies. I know that traditional Chinese health practices avoided surgery, but didn't children in China have tonsillitis and appendicitis? How were they treated?"

Surgery and acupuncture care for tonsillitis and appendicitis with wonderful results. Since the throat acts as the thru-way for the Lung and the Stomach, abundant Heat from these Organs ascends to the tonsils. Heat is the culprit for appendicitis too. It stagnates in the Large Intestine and generates a condition called "Intestinal Abscess." In either case, needling and herbs should clear the Heat. But if there is no response, it is time to see a surgeon.

How does acupuncture treat alternating diarrhea and constipation?

"As a grandmother, I see my grandchildren suffering from the same digestive problems I remember with my children. First it's diarrhea then constipation. Frequent pains in the tummy and nausea with stuffy nose and coughing are other complaints. Just as they told me years ago, pediatricians tell my daughter that the kids have allergies or a virus. Even with medication these ailments continue. You would think medicine could do something from one generation to the next."

Problems with eating are most common among children, and all part of growing up. During this period, the body must metabolize large amounts of food by a digestive system that has to mature as well. The symptoms you mention fit into a familiar pattern. Chinese medicine calls it "accumulation disorder." Some weak Organs and hard-to-digest meals cause ingested food to pile up and decay inside the body. Heat and blockages soon follow with pains and nausea.

Organ disharmony mainly involves the Spleen and Stomach. Since they regulate dryness and lubrication, coughs and nasal congestion become related problems. Acupuncture helps by opening obstructions and by strengthening the Spleen and Stomach.

More easily consumed food consists of preparations cooked well and served with white rice. It helps when you avoid large amounts of raw and heavily rich items.

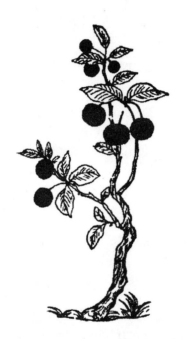

Litchi fruits (Nephilium litchi)

5

Diet

Countries all over the world serve Chinese food. In China and everywhere else with diverse ethnic restaurants, you cannot miss the specialties of Canton, Beijing, Szechwan and Hunan. People love to consume these Oriental delicacies, whether to eat in, take out or prepare at home.

Few people realize that Chinese cuisine contains recipes that are designed for reasons of health and in accordance with the principles of Chinese medicine. There are Yin and Yang ingredients and seasonings designed to nourish Essence and Blood. Different dishes are composed to go with different seasons and different climates. With Chinese cuisine it is possible to eat to gain energy to sustain and strengthen body functions. Like the rest of the culture, China's way of making meals developed from ancient traditions.

According to Chinese medicine, what is the role of diet in maintaining health?

"Western science has analyzed food substance thoroughly. We know all about vitamins, minerals, protein, fat and carbohydrates. Also, we calculate daily requirements and understand calories. Dietitians and doctors recommend special dishes to prevent and accommodate diseases. So what does Chinese medicine have to add to our knowledge about food and health?"

There are two types of Qi energy in your body that need to be nourished: Inherited Qi and Acquired Qi. Inherited Qi (which comes from one's parents and ancestors and must last a lifetime) involves inherited Essence (Jing) and Spirit (Shen), the duration of both of which is maintained by diet. Acquired Qi relies directly on daily replenishing through food and drink and air. In other words, instead of discussing nutrition in terms of chemical nutrients, acupuncture considers your internal system of Qi energy as it is received from parents at birth and afterwards from the soil, lakes and air.

What you eat, of course, has nutritional value based on its chemical composition. But in addition to evaluating this kind of nutritional value, Chinese medine can influence your diet by assessing food in relation to your internal environment to insure that it remain in harmony with changes outside. The preparation of a health-conscious Chinese meal takes into account Yin and Yang, time of the year, climate, conditions of residence and individual temperament. Hot, cold, damp or dry conditions in varied proportions exist around you and within you. Food alters your internal, bodily environment just as weather, climate and conditions of residence change the world outside. Both must be watched so that food preparation can be adjusted as conditions, both internal and external, change. Awareness of Yin and Yang can guide us in creating balanced diets. Chinese cooking and kitchen skills include ways of understanding foods in terms of Yin and Yang, the Five Elements, as well as the other categories, so that food preparation can be correlated with internal and external conditions.

Haven't countries outside of China set the table with good, balanced meals?

Though unaware of how their cultural cuisines really do regulate and balance energy, many nations throughout the world cook in accordance with what in fact are acupuncture principles. The Chinese culinary health science that understands how flavors are related to the Five Elements goes far to explain why people eat as they do, taking sustenance according to the appeal of flavors.

How does the Chinese understanding of the nutritional content of food compare to that of Western medicine, and how does this affect dietary choices?

Never in human history has food undergone such analysis as in the modern laboratory. We measure exact amounts for everything. Labels tell us what vitamins and minerals we eat; they inform us of a product's fat, carbohydrate, protein and cholesterol content, and how many calories it delivers. Western nutritional science also gives advice on daily requirements and recommends special diets. In reading the fine print, we can learn of the artificial substances these foods contain, and if we inform ourselves from scientifically reliable sources, we can learn of their harmful effects.

Chinese nutritional science, in contrast, reveals the Yin and Yang and the taste category of foods. It advises that, in order to harmonize with nature, we should eat with the forces of nature: the weather, territory, and a person's Qi all should set the stage for the dining scene.

Regardless of dinner plans and the make-up of each course, it's the digestive Qi that must metabolize solids and acquired Qi. Under the microscope and in the test tube, food may appear wholesome. But the capability of your particular body to break down those enriched morsels has much bearing on the nutritional effect of the meal. The weak or the very aged do not present the same potential to consume and digest as the young and the robust, so the same food will have different nutritional value for different people. For example, brown rice has more food-value than white when analyzed chemically, but white rice is easier to digest.

What are the basic dietary principles according to Chinese medicine?

After negative emotions and harmful invasions from the external environment, the most important factor in causing disease is poor diet.

Here are a few Chinese dietary principles:

- Chinese medicine is very concerned with the distinction between Hot and Cold in relation to food, and in general advises against cold food. The main reason is that the Triple Warmer — the complex of Organ-energy systems that is responsible for the assimilation and distribution of Qi energy — requires Heat to function properly. Trapped Cold within the gastrointestinal tract causes symptoms for which the Western diagnoses would be bacterial, viral, or parasitic infections and ulcers.

- Lack of diversity in diet in general automatically suggests unhealthy eating. Variety in diet should be dictated by the seasonal availability of fresh food, the Elemental association of the season, local weather conditions, and individual constitution.

- Binges on large amounts of rich and fatty delicacies harm the two Organs of digestion: the Spleen and Stomach. Too much of such food causes particles to accumulate and stagnate. This generates excessive Heat and in some people may cause diabetes. Excessive alcohol will contribute to and aggravate this tendency.

- Although Chinese provinces cook with and without meat, vegetarianism offers wonderful health benefits. With dishes derived from Oriental cuisines rich in soy bean inventions such as tofu, there is no danger of an insufficient intake of protein.

• Whole fresh fish has long been a Chinese dinner staple. But, compared to the United States, China shows relatively small amounts of animal protein annually consumed per person. The amount of vegetable protein consumed by the average Chinese person accordingly far exceeds the intake of the average American.

• The dominance of vegetables and grains is recommended to allow for body harmony.

• In general, dietary choice should be determined by individual need. Any acupuncture practitioner or dietitian familiar with Chinese use of the Five Elements and the forces of nature in connection with cooking can give advice on specifics.

How is the Five Element System used to determine correct Diet?

The Chinese categorize food according to the same "Five Element" system that they use to understand the Organ system and the processes of the external world. Foods are understood according to the five "Flavors" that they contain; each Flavor is associated with an element, a season, a color, an Organ, and other things *(See the chart on pages 52-53).*

The Qi of each of the Five Flavors improves the Qi of the Five Organs, which sustain the Essence and Spirit. To understand the influences of the Flavors, one must know the benefits for each Organ and the dangers from excesses and deficiencies. Foods are also categorized in regard to Yin and Yang for balanced blending.

Let's look at each of these tastes in order:

Sour

Sour relates to Wood, the vibrant green burst of spring, and the vitality of Wind. This phase of existence is associated with the sourness of unripe fruit and the fermentation of vinegar. As when spring *wind dries* winter's melted snow and scatters irrigating water, the acid substances regulate excess body fluid and toughen the skin. The ability of that bit of lemon to activate water lets us enjoy lemonade, tea, and fish.

One of several chores for the Liver, the Wood Organ, is to spread energy. In the Cycle of Organs, the Liver precedes the Heart. Therefore, consuming "sour" food enhances the Liver's ability to care for a slow-paced Heart. Sour stops diarrhea and running noses, and relieves Lung congestion and weak dermatological tissues. In accordance with these principles, even in the West, lemon and vinegar have long been used as folk-medicines to break up colds.

Nations in Eastern Europe traditionally ferment and pickle their food. Dining on sauerkraut, sauerbraten, pickled beets and cucumbers brings a little bit of inner spring during the autumn months, fortifies the skin and heart, and, incidentally, acts as a good adjustment for the inhabitants of a landscape of clear, fresh water, rivers and lakes. Vinegar, in addition to belonging to the sour category, also exemplifies the bitter, which enhances its benefits in treating indigestion, bleeding disorders and toxins. However, beware of damage to the Liver from too much sour ingestion. Also, abstain from sourness in the presence of tendon disorders, as the Liver controls tendons and this would aggravate the problem.

Bitter

Bitter is associated with the Heart and the Element of Fire. It can warm the body's interior, remove toxins, and bring a cooling effect, since the bitter influence dries heat-infested dampness. Both bitter and sour flavors nurture the Liver, the Wood Element, which accordingly improves the Heart, the Fire Element, as Wood nourishes Fire.

Lots of non-sweetened coffee, tea, and hot chocolate will get you through the winter. In freezing weather, you might also try putting condiments made from horseradish on your food. Flavors mix to blend a palatable dish. Stuffing ourselves with too much of one taste can harm Organ energy. For example, an abundance of bitterness withers the skin and hair and weakens the bone. But in proper dosages, bitter foods are very medicinal. They warm the body with the red Fire of summer, which promotes circulation and strength. The Fire Element Organ, the Heart, desires these substances. Residents in cold climates feel the glow from a strong condiment or a cup of hot chocolate. But even there, or during the winter in more temperate places, it is helpful to balance the devouring of hot drying staples with a cooler moistening snack.

Sweet

The sweet taste of honey, ripe fruit, grains and meat connect with Spleen-Stomach, the yellow Element of Earth and the period of late summer or Indian summer, when humidity *stagnates* and we experience a coming together in the *stillness* of the year. After the formative spring and blossoming summer, a maturity endures for awhile, sustaining the peak of nature's creative forces. Sweet it is before the autumn harvest and the fall of the leaves.

Dairy products are categorized as moist and sweet. In the cow, milk completes a process that the ingested green grass of spring began. Chinese diet tends to avoid dairy products, in contrast to that of the West, perhaps in anticipation of recent medical research that shows milk to be the source of allergies, excessive mucus, and fat build-up.

Flavors as well as times of day can be associated with Yin and Yang. Food can in this way be used to balance qualities of time. For instance, any warm sunny Yang morning merits a glass of Yin fruit juice--whether sweet and sour orange or apple or less sour pear.

Combining flavors combines effects. Folk medicine uses sour Wood Element vinegar to disperse cogestion, but the blending of vinegar with the sweet Earth Element honey can calm coughs and inflammation.

Food substances possess inherent traits. The manner of preparation, however, may alter these basic characters. Hot sweet foods instill *insulation* for warmth, or *store* heavy dampness. Oven-baked or oven-roasted meat *retains* fat and counters the Yin chills of the wintry North. Broiling beef on a grill or rotating it on a spit before an open fire eliminates grease, which makes it more appealing and beneficial at summer barbecues. Yin dairy moistens in arid climates. As milk hardens into cheese, it leans toward Yang.

Swiss cheese accommodates the *dry* mountain air of Switzerland, with a touch of Yang for warmth. Desert regions that long for the "Land of Milk and Honey," use light dairy products that offer cool refreshment. Thorough studies of eating with regard to various surroundings exist and form a complex subject, which is as important for correct diet as knowledge of the chemistry of nutrients.

Spicy

Acrid tastes are associated with dehydrated autumn harvests. This flavor is associated with the aeration of Lungs and the whiteness of metal. The Element is Metal; however, an extended understanding of this flavor involves the element Air as well.

Damp, tropical regions all over the world have developed pungent cuisines like those of Mexico, New Orleans, India or Szechwan, China. Unlike the north, whose lakes and seas give it a cool and thin Yin feature, the tropics swamp the land with hot and heavy bodies of water.

Strong, spicy seasonings dry the body's interior to create harmony with extensive wetlands. Foods using the Sour flavor have a draining effect in airy, wet internal territories, but it is not enough for rain forest areas.

If your menu contains numerous drying ingredients in an already dry area, expect dehydration. Too much dryness lingers within you. But oil acts as a lubricant. By tradition and intuition, Mediterranean and desert nations cook with Yin oil to soothe the scorch of the hot, arid sun. Oil is fine, but the excessive use of spices in such places may produce dehydration. A moderate amount of pungent seasoning, however, is good to help balance heavy, oily, fatty, or greasy recipes.

Salty

The following set of symptoms belongs to a person suffering from an imbalance of Kidney Qi, the Organ associated with the Flavor, salty: Sore low back and aching knees that feel better when swimming in salt water; ringing in the ears, arthritis, and a tendency for lump formation (nodules) under the skin. This person, incidentally, tends to choose black colors for the clothes he wears.

The flavor of salt, the color black, ringing in the ears and pain in the low back and knees belong to the Water Element, winter, and the Kidney Organ. The relief that comes from swimming in the ocean is caused by the fact that the Ocean's water and salt nourish deficiencies of this Organ.

A dietary supplement of salt can also help restore these deficiencies, but salt will cause harm if there is a blood disorder or swelling due to a kidney infection.

Lumps form under the skin after Qi stagnates. The responsibility for "dispersion" (which overcomes stagnation) belongs to the Liver. In the cycle of energy, the Kidney provides energy to the Liver. Therefore, caring for the Kidney aids the Liver. Similarly, if the Kidney is deficient in Qi, the Liver may fail to perform its duties. In accordance with this line of reasoning, Chinese medicine treats congealed masses with naturally formed salt from food and some herbs of the sea. Needling to stimulate Kidney and Liver Qi helps to dissipate stagnation.

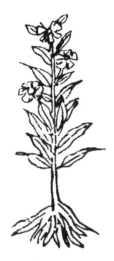

Rough Gentian

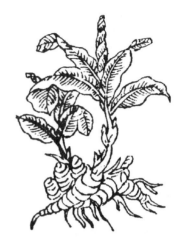

Turmeric

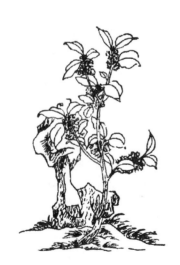

Cinnamon

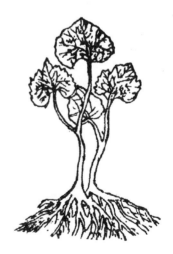

Wild Ginger

Is a vegan-vegetarian diet more healthy than one that includes meat and dairy products?

"For many years I have had vegetarian habits. I think it's much healthier not to take in all that animal fat, which is bad for the heart and arteries. Also, I don't drink much milk, the so-called perfect food, nor candy or ice cream. I do eat plenty of fruit though. I have meat-eating and milk-eating friends who are heavier than I and who suffer from allergies and frequent colds. Otherwise, they're in good health. I feel the chills of winter more than they; still, isn't a vegan-vegetarian diet more healthy than one that includes meat and dairy products?"

Under many circumstances, meat and milk do their damage. Underactive Spleen energy prohibits absorption of excess Dampness from animal products, which leads to disease. A lactose-free, vegetarian way of life may yield healthier nourishment. Weighty individuals carrying around the cumulative hot moisture of fat, certainly do not need more of the same during humid summer weather. Of various food requirement factors, the most important truly concerns the physical make-up of the individual, the climate where he or she lives, and the weather.

How can I apply the principles of Chinese cooking as a foundation for my day-to-day meals?

Without complete familiarity with all the ways to design a perfect meal, you still may apply general knowledge of nature's forces. But remember that dosages have relevance. Not enough water, we die of thirst; too much water, we drown. Blend ingredients for the time of day, season, and your internal health status. You will eat differently in the cool of the summer's evening than under the hot noon sun.

My guidelines for interpreting the cuisines of different cultures stem from a creative application of acupuncture concepts. To me it makes sense to eat energy balanced meals anywhere, anytime.

By this logic, China cooks according to the province and the season. Peking duck has the grease and fat appropriate for northern winters. The southern damp areas of Szechwan and Hunan use seasoning with drying herbs. There's the right food for every land and the right mixture for every season.

Why do the Chinese eat white rice instead of brown?

"Husking the brown strips it of important vitamins and minerals. My doctor recommended white rice for a digestive problem. Someone told me that the old Chinese nobility ate white rice and the rest of the population copied them. Yet, doesn't nutrition take priority over prestige in dining?"

Most of China's cuisine calls for white rice, not because of the chemistry of vitamins, minerals, protein, fat, carbohydrates or digestive enzymes and certainly not to imitate royalty. White rice is eaten to help maintain balance. The catalyst for *normalizing* is white rice. It balances Yin with Yang; it neutralizes the powers and after-effects of tastes; finally, it digests more easily than the brown rice.

My grandparents seem to be in good shape for their age but their diet is horrendous. How is this possible?

"My grandparents are slender and active and have a happy disposition, but their diet is incredible: boiled hot dogs and baked beans are a favorite. I cannot convince them that heat destroys vitamins and garden salads retain elements of nutrition. They do eat a lot of fruit, however. In comparison, I keep myself in top form by aerobics, lots of salads and white meat or fish on occasion. Is there a generation gap?"

At different points in life, the body changes its needs. The hot Yang of youth feels comfortable with cool refreshments. As aging reduces the fire, the elderly—particularly those on the thin side—savor warmth from cooked and fatty foods. Your grandparents get plenty of vitamins from their fruit, and their apparent positive outlook allows their Organs to function well. They seem fine to me.

I have been diagnosed with gastritis—the prelude to an ulcer, but I don't feel I am under stress. Can acupuncture help me?

"I have always had a good hearty diet with very little junk food. A year ago I felt pain above my stomach, lost my appetite and became nauseous. The diagnosis came after a barium X ray. My doctor advised bland meals. I followed his instructions, but I still get the pain and nauseousness. I used to eat more salads; now I feel better with warm food and hot drinks. I do not understand why I should be sick if I always ate nourishing food. My friends say it's stress, yet I handle stress very well. Can acupuncture help me?"

Your relief from warmer beverages and food indicates Cold in the Stomach, perhaps due to an abundance of raw salads. Cold can also invade from the atmosphere. Acupuncture treatments would offer you a correction by heating and regulating the Spleen and Stomach, while the Cold makes an exit. Much of the fault centers on your Organ energy, not your diet. Until you find an acupuncturist, however, stick with some warm supplements at mealtime.

What can acupuncture do about anorexia?

"Recently I was diagnosed as anorexic. My weight had dropped considerably, since I do not have much appetite. There's dryness in my mouth and I experience gas and constipation. My family physician recommended psychological counseling, as I am a habitual worrier."

Western medicine will interpret your symptoms as a severe nervous condition. Although in Chinese medicine worry is associated with the Stomach-Spleen, your dry mouth and constipation give the message that you are suffering from a Yin-Yang imbalance. When the lubricating, wet Yin falls, an empty Fire Yang takes over. In your case, you have deficient Yin of the Stomach. A thorough acupuncture examination, including pulse and tongue evaluations, will present more detailed information. Then an increase of Yin with acupuncture treatments should restore your health. Regulating Organ energy also will strengthen your emotions.

Loss of appetite could occur from numerous sources. That's why in acupuncture every symptom holds diagnostic importance. Where the West will concentrate on food intake, organ structure and digestive enzymes, the East examines Qi and disparities of Yin and Yang. Metabolic Organs as well as internal environmental disturbances of Cold, Hot, Damp or Dry merit attention. In addition to all this, blockages and stagnation may be causing Stomach and Intestinal disorders.

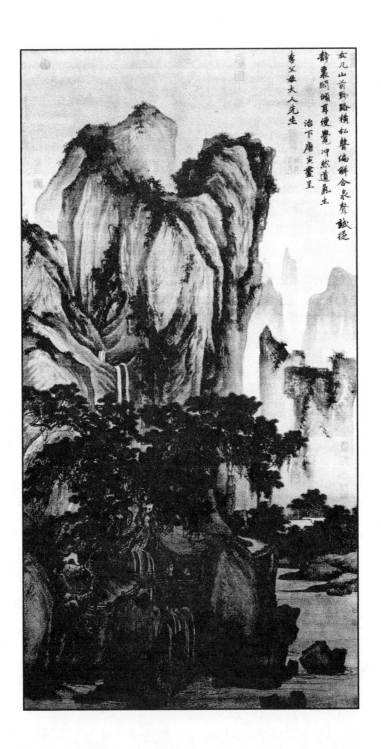

女几山前野路橫松聲偏稱合泉聲　誠傳

靜裏閒傾耳便覺沖然道氣生

治下唐寅畫呈

嚴父母大人先生

6

Medical Emergencies

Can acupuncture treat physical accidents and emergencies—broken bones, or gunshot wounds for instance?

Western medicine with its paramedics and rescue squads does very well in providing immediate care for accident victims. Historically, much of this aspect of our medicine grew from handling military emergencies and applying the techniques developed there to civilian crisis situations. Chinese medicine similarly developed military applications which can be applied to accidents back home.

In Chinese battles, needles and herbs came to the rescue while bandaging injuries. The first article I wrote on acupuncture for a medical journal was titled "Treatment Of Emergencies With Acupuncture." My illustrations showed how combined Western-Eastern treatments help to save lives. Personally, I have come to the aid of many sufferers in crises with acupuncture and have prevented disasters.

The East and West offer different ways of assessment and different methods of treatment. Both systems work. In China, acupuncture manages emergency room problems. Integration of acupuncture in the crisis facilities of American hospitals would save many lives.

(LEFT) *T'ang Yin*, Whispering Pines on a Mountain Path. (*Undated, Ca. 1516*)

Can acupuncture treat shock?

"In first aid classes we're taught that shock results from decreased blood circulation in the external parts of the body. Loss of blood results in inadequate oxygen. That's why the shock victim has cold, moist, pale and bluish skin. Instructions tell us to keep the patient warm, elevate the legs a little, stop any bleeding and make sure of an open airway for breathing. In a hospital setting, fluid replacement and medication may be helpful. I would like to know how acupuncture treats shock?"

Shock is classified by causes and symptoms. Your description of it is accurate; however, where Western doctors see deficient blood, acupuncturists also recognize energy loss. When Yin Blood drops down, Yang Qi goes with it. As acupuncture replenishes exhausted Yang, Yin also boosts up to restore Blood. The stimulation of certain acupuncture points will accomplish this. Needling techniques raise Yang and Qi, but also elicit actions to calm the Spirit and regulate the Heart. The restoration of balanced Qi-Blood circulation then normalizes the ill-effects of shock.

Western first aid in fact actually does influence energy systems. A warm blanket causes the retention of Yang. Raising the legs and preventing further blood loss holds the Blood with the Qi. An unobstructed breath will inhale Acquired Qi for systemic benefits.

What does acupuncture do for simple fainting?

Medical science in the West usually sees reduced blood flow through the brain as the culprit in fainting. Slow heart rates curb circulation. Immediate care rests the fainter on a flat surface. As a rule, heart examinations should follow an episode of unconsciousness.

Oriental medicine, in such cases, looks for disturbances in the Qi, which hold back Blood from one's head. Overwork and emotional problems cause *rebellion* amongst certain forms of Qi. Acupuncture steps in to straighten out the turmoil and strengthen the weak circulation.

How would acupuncture take a person out of a coma? Can needles restore consciousness?

When doctors who have been trained in the Western school of medicine find someone in a coma, they look for several causes. A tumor of the brain or spinal cord, especially a blood tumor called a hematoma, may produce unconsciousness. Other reasons may involve head injuries, cerebral bleeding, infection, lack of oxygen, poison, epilepsy and psychological problems. Unknown causes prompt the attending physician to order tests from the lab and x-ray departments. Immediate life-saving steps call for CPR (cardiopulmonary resuscitation), provision of an airway for breathing and stoppage of bleeding if present. Routinely, hospitals administer oxygen and fluid replacement. In a situation with diabetic patients, examiners must consider the difference between too much sugar in the blood (diabetic coma) or too much insulin (insulin shock). The giving of insulin or sugar will then regulate the hormonal imbalance. Whatever the cause, attendees periodically check rates of the pulse, blood pressure, temperature and respiration.

In emergencies, as with all disorders, successful recoveries depend on knowing what disturbs the internal environment and how acupuncture points direct change. According to Chinese medicine, the above causes all have another dimension that relates to the Heart and Pericardium, Hot or Cold Mucus, and blockages. Heat can drop into the Pericardium (the area surrounding the heart); Hot Mucus can obstruct the Pericardium, or Cold Mucus can "mist" the Heart openings.

In Chinese medicine, we have to talk about the afflicted Organs and their detrimental atmosphere. Since the Heart controls the blood vessels and blood circulation and also shelters the mind, we can see connections between bleeding, hematomas and mental states. As the protector of the Heart and the circulator of Kidney Yang Qi, the Pericardium pushes energy to every part of the body. If these Organs can't do their jobs, there's trouble.

To treat coma with acupuncture, we select points on the basis of the Chinese understanding of patterned conditions. Mainly, we want to disperse the Heat or Cold, clear the senses, clear the Brain, calm the Spirit, eliminate Phlegm and strengthen the Heart. A twirl of the needle through chosen spots on the skin accomplishes these tasks. Some points need to be pierced and bled a drop to drain congested channels.

Another difference between Western and Chinese medicine in regard to coma is this: where Western medicine differentiates separate comatose disorders, acupuncture groups symptoms by similarities. For instance, Hot Phlegm that agitates the Heart can yield brain inflammation, epilepsy or stroke. In a like manner, emergency acupuncture points and emergency drugs restore consciousness, no matter what the cause. Once consciousness is restored, special points or drugs perform their unique actions as indicated. In China, acupuncture manages emergency room problems. As a repeated and valuable suggestion, the integration of acupuncture in the crisis facilities of American hospitals could save many lives.

Is acupuncture compatible with Western lifesaving measures? Are there certain acupuncture points that can be used in an emergency?

Acupuncture goes hand in hand with revival medications, CPR (cardio-pulmonary rescucitation), bag-mask oxygen respiration, and other such lifesaving methods. Proper needle manipulation may reduce the need both for severe, rescuing jolts to the patient and for surgery.

Pressing your finger against specific emergency points while moving the skin back and forth or in a circle can give valuable first aid. Of course, nothing substitutes for the thorough awareness of energy systems and acupuncture points possessed by needle-trained acupuncturists; however, there are certain techniques that, like the Heimlich maneuver, are easy to learn and may save lives. Here are a few examples:

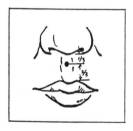

Jan-chung

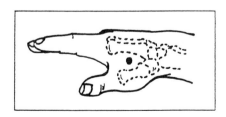

Ho-ku

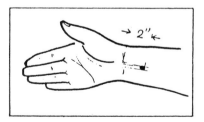

Nei-kuan

A commonly used point for restoring consciousness, whatever the cause of its loss, can be found one-third of the way down the groove from the nasal septum or two-thirds of the way up from the upper lip below the nose. This point is called Governing Vessel 26, since the point is on the Governing Vessel—a special channel that ascends the back and goes over the head. Stimulation of GV 26 (Jan-chung) regulates energy through the head and brain. This point can also be used to treat extreme allergic reactions, collapse, coma, debilitated breathing, epilepsy, fainting, heat exhaustion, hysteria, motion sickness and seizures. Dig your fingernail into the middle of the "mustache" area below the nose and you may just awake an out-of-it victim!

To relieve dizziness, nosebleed, throat blockage, or headache, hold the patient's hand and press your finger into the fleshy bulge on the other side of the crease from the base of the thumb. The skin protrudes here when the thumb and index finger close together. Add support in the palm area directly underneath. The Chinese name for this point is "Meeting Valleys" (Ho-ku) since the skin depressions inside the thumb and index finger unite to project the point location. Situated on the Hand Large Intestine Meridian, it has the designation of Large Intestine 4. However, do not use this point on pregnant women.

You can buy a flexible bracelet with a small ball on the inner side that curbs motion sickness, whether in boats, cars and planes. Also, morning sickness during pregnancy lessens with this band. The affect stems from the pressure of the ball into an acupuncture point.

On the underside of the arm between two tendons, you will find a spot two thumb widths back from the farthest wrist crease. Applying pressure here will treat chest-related emergencies— asthma and lung dysfunctions, chest pain, heart palpitations, hiccough, stomach pain, and (the little bracelet ball will do this too), nausea and vomiting. This is Pericardium 6 (Nei-kuan) and a good point to know, especially for children and the elderly.

Can acupuncture be used for a drowning victim, unconscious but still alive in a hospital bed?

Make every effort to insist that an acupuncturist joins the medical team. After resuscitation, needle stimulation clears obstructions chiefly in the Heart and Brain. At the same time, the acupuncturist will normalize the Lungs and Blood circulation to restore consciousness.

How can acupuncture help a broken leg or sprained wrist?

Physical trauma tears soft tissue and fractures bone. Immobilizing the inflicted area with splints or casts supports the healing mechanism and allows the body to cure itself. If prescribed, physical therapy and chiropractic adjustments facilitate rehabilitation in follow-up treatments.

In Chinese medicine, injury to an extremity of the body means interference of energy flow through Channels. Acupuncture treatments can supplement Western methods to restore normal circulation of Qi, which in turn improves the Blood's ability to nourish the injured or healing areas.

Can acupuncture help with accidents that strike the neck and spine?

Yes. By the same course of therapy that moves Qi to damaged parts, acupuncture treats any injury, which includes the neck and spine.

Are there ways to *see* the repair of energy?

Yes. This has been demonstrated by Kirlian photography before and after trauma. This method for photographing unique patterns of light around living objects shows the return of normal body-energy after treatment, by actually displaying the "aura" of "Protective Qi."

Is acupuncture most helpful at the onset of a symptom or during recuperation?

Acupuncture applies relief at both times. Time-proven methods cover a wide scope of crucial situations, from a bleeding nose to hastening delayed labor before delivery. Added to rescue operations, acupuncture will be a lifesaver. Rehabilitation employs acupuncture to restore damaged tissue and function. Through methods of unblocking congestion and of directing Qi and Blood where needed, patients often recover quite rapidly.

7

Acupuncture and Aids

Is acupuncture the answer to AIDS?

The crises spreads with still unpredictable consequences. A few years ago, many thought that AIDS stayed in the communities of homosexual men, intravenous addicts and the far reaches of Africa. Now the disease plagues male-female couples, infants and teenagers. Blood transfusions and pregnant mothers transmit HIV. Western medicine hopes to discover a vaccine. But perhaps the answers lie not in *destroying* viruses, but instead in *restoring* immunity to ravaged immune systems and strengthening a sick internal environment with acupuncture and herbs.

What are the major differences between traditional Chinese and modern Western approaches to the treatment of AIDS?

How each form of medicine takes responsibility for dealing with the AIDS epidemic reveals the innermost principles of the two health care systems. Interestingly, the very Western terms that name this disease correspond to important terms within Chinese medicine. AIDS is a name made up of the first letters of the words: Acquired ImmunoDeficiency Syndrome. Patients *acquire* harmful conditions, because of *deficiencies* in *immunity* that result in a *syndrome* or pattern of symptoms. The letters HIV stand for Human Immunodeficiency Virus—a name that suggests typically Western medical ideas, focusing on a *visible* virus. However, in spite of press coverage that would suggest that there is total agreement on the subject, not everyone in Western medicine accepts the hypothesis that HIV is the cause of AIDS.

Acupuncture cares for AIDS patients with the *same* age-old diagnostic methods that it has used for centuries. The symptoms of AIDS are not new, therefore the treatment is not new. Since Western science looks for viral causes and since it first learned of the HIV virus very recently, it seeks for a new method to handle the epidemic.

Acupuncture therapy directs its attention to symptom relief and immunity enhancement. As damaging heat, wind and dampness drain away in response to treatment, the internal environment undergoes change. Yin and Yang develop better linkages. Organs, Qi energy, and Blood gain more strength. Stagnation moves so that blockages clear.

Western medicine prescribes antiviral drugs like AZT as research perseveres in its search for a vaccine to prevent infection by HIV. Complications of bacterial infections and tumors receive the standard care of antibiotics, surgery and chemotherapy. Unfortunately, antibiotics cannot effectively treat a viral disease, and AZT cannot destroy HIV but only hamper its reproduction and may further damage the immune system along the way.

What is a virus and how is it treated in Western medicine?

Biology considers viruses to be the smallest living objects in existence. Viruses are parasites, totally dependent on their victims or hosts for survival. Several sicknesses traced to viral infections no longer have the chance to become epidemics, thanks to vaccines that produce immunity. These include polio, rabies, and yellow fever. Due to the success of past vaccines, Western science thinks it should be possible to find one for HIV.

Do viruses possess the energy of Qi?

Yes, all life has Qi, but disease-related viruses are associated with toxic energy.

Is there a chance that AIDS occurs without a virus, or from other causes?

According to the understanding of Chinese medicine, AIDS actually has a non-viral origin. The abnormal or pathological Qi provides room for HIV. Normal Qi is Qi that performs a function in maintaining health. The state of well-being itself opposes abnormal Qi, the destructive powers that attack the body.

What is the energetic basis for the treatment of AIDS?

Quite simply, acupuncture seeks to support the normal Qi and expel disease-producing influences. It drives stronger carriers of energy to push and fuel up the weaker. Meanwhile it throws aside dangerous obstacles. The Western attitude of crushing invading pathogens with deadly weapons like AZT, which is known to weaken the immune system, contradicts the Chinese application. Since violent therapy strikes healthy bodily systems as well as diseased, the normal Qi can be damaged by it.

Since Western medicine understands the immune system pretty well, what in addition can acupuncture offer?

Western medicine understands immunity as a system for counterattacking intruders. Invading bacteria and viruses contain antigens (specific, toxic, foreign substances) which act on the body to stimulate the production of "antibodies"—molecules specifically evolved to fight specific, toxic, foreign substances.

A different dimension of our being comes into play when acupuncture studies AIDS and immunity. The presence of toxins in Channels, excesses and deficiencies in Organ energy, Yin-Yang imbalances, and negative qualities of Blood and Qi all indicate a susceptibility to poor health—what in Western medicine is understood as immune deficiency."

The acupuncture distinction between inborn energy and acquired energy is similar to the Western distinction between acquired and "natural" immunity. The process by which antigens stimulate the production of antibodies is similar to the way, in the acupuncture conception, acquired energy produces protective energy. Inborn resistance, called "natural" immunity by Western medicine, compares to inherited energy.

The best way to understand AIDS is by combining Chinese and Western understanding of the details of the functioning of the immune system. The best way to treat it is with acupuncture techniques for clearing toxins, nourishing Blood and Qi, adjusting the Organs, and balancing Yin and Yang.

How do acupuncturists treat AIDS?

With needling and with herbs. Abnormal Qi mainly injures three Organ energy fields: the Kidney, the Spleen with its partner the Stomach, and the Lung. Identifiable symptoms follow Organ-related disruptions. From a depletion of Lung Qi, there arises breathing difficulties such as asthma, allergies, and frequent colds. Diminishing Spleen Yang, complicated with excess internal dampness, causes digestive problems, lack of appetite, nausea, and diarrhea, plus moist skin eruptions. Kidney losses result in general weakness.

Treatments reverse the destructive process as in other diseases with the same symptoms. Moreover, special effort is made with AIDS victims to try to evacuate bad Qi and poisons, while normal Organ Qi and Essence (Jing) are given a chance to replenish themselves.

How does acupuncture needling rehabilitate AIDS patients?

Needling acupuncture points and applying herbal heat stimulate a wide range of reactions. Documented improvements in the immune system continue to appear in patients' records, which show increased red and macrophage white blood cells. Acupuncture techniques strengthen each of the three Organ systems usually weakened by the AIDS viral associations (Lung, Spleen, Kidney) as the case may be, which in turn relieves associated problems.

Also, acupuncture brings down fever, calms negative emotions, stops pain and itching, and expels the harmful pollutants.

Where are case studies on acupuncture and AIDS published?

Here are two important references: In the March 1987 issue of *The American Journal of Acupuncture,* Dr. Naomi Rabinowitz presented the important paper: "Acupuncture and the AIDS Epidemic: Reflections on the Treatment of 200 Patients in Four Years." In it she combines explanations of the disease process according to acupuncture logic with details from her medical background. The article describes such improvements as reduced physical and emotional symptoms, and the prevention of further debilitation in patients treated for AIDS with acupuncture.

In the June 1988 issue of this same journal, Dr. Michael Smith's paper, "AIDS: Results of Chinese Medical Treatments Show Frequent Symptom Relief and Some Apparent Long-Term Remissions," reports positive results from both needles and oral herbs.

Do you believe that solutions to the AIDS epidemic will be found in Chinese herbs?

Yes, because already Chinese herbal remedies have improved conditions for AIDS patients.

How were herbs for treating AIDS found?

Epidemics and plagues have occurred in both Chinese and Western history. During periods of mass disease, Chinese doctors experimented with herbs to bring relief. It turns out that many of the AIDS symptoms correspond to symptoms studied by Chinese doctors during these times. Chinese medicine had also achieved success in finding herbal remedies for rebuilding strength in cancer patients.

A search in these already successful resources found suitable ingredients for treating AIDS.

How is acupuncture AIDS research being conducted today?

For almost twenty years, the Fuzheng Therapy Coordinating Group in China has done extensive research with herbs for cancer. Due to similarities in weaknesses between cancer and AIDS, its findings apply to deficiencies in both diseases. The word "Fuzheng" refers to the support of normal Qi.

In an international conference on immunity held in Beijing in 1983, the presentation of effects from a certain root and a certain fruit motivated production to make the compound available in the United States. The compound also contained a therapeutic mushroom, which both China and Japan had been experimenting with for its enhancement properties.

In America, most of the work to develop natural therapies to enhance the immune system takes place on the West Coast.

American herbalists are developing their art and science in conjunction with Oriental institutions. In 1986, the Immune Enhancement Project centralized its office of operations at Berkeley, California. Since then, statistical studies have constantly demonstrated progressive improvements in AIDS sufferers through the use of herbs.

The Chinese Medicinal Materials Research Centre at the Chinese University of Hong Kong serves as a gigantic resource center for documentation, which has been gathered over years of investigation. At the Arnold Arboretum of Harvard University, scientific studies offer valuable facts about Chinese plants. Jointly, the

Oriental Healing Arts Institute of Long Beach, California and the Brion Research Institute of Taiwan provide formulas and information on recent findings. Throughout China, the Academy of Traditional Chinese Medicine assembles patient data from herbal therapies. These outstanding bodies of research and compilers of academic material have published numerous books and journals.

This sea of knowledge is being organized by the Institute of Traditional Medicine (ITM) in Portland, Oregon. Its books, videos, and subscribed publications continue to educate practitioners of Oriental medicine. Most of my research for this chapter comes from ITM sources, in particular, the book *Chinese Herbal Therapies For Immune Disorders*.

In the 1980s, Dr. Subhuti Dharmanada, ITM's director, author and herbalist authority, together with another herbalist, Reese Smith, prepared guidelines for HIV treatments. ITM established the Immune Enhancement Project and the work never stops.

How do herbs for AIDS differ from drugs for AIDS?

Nature gives us herbs for food and medicine. By implication herbal medicine *is* food. It's available from plants, animals and minerals. Secrets of herbal vegetation hide in fruits, roots, seeds, leaves, bark, stems and flowers. Chinese medicine is based on human responses to the herb. The science of herbology works with natural forces to solve AIDS. It regulates energy to remove the unwanted.

Western pharmacology also matches substances with reactions.

In place of directing attention to the Chinese understanding of Qi, drug companies analyze chemistry in relation to the composition of the body and the AIDS virus. Whether we derive the medicine from laboratory synthesis or from an altered natural extraction, we just cannot look at it as God's gift to humanity. Instead, this is man's invention to control pathology.

Has there been any progress in AIDS research with improved mixtures of herbs?

The Oriental Healing Arts Institute's initial compound, Astra 8, strengthens Organs and expels toxins for popular usage. An up-to-date formula, Composition-A, produced by the Institute for Traditional Medicine, provides many actions to nourish, tonify and release harmful elements. Depending on symptoms, other herbs can supplement these two remedies. An injectable herb known as Compound Q only attaches to cells infected with HIV. Researchers are still investigating its potential.

Selections of herbs accommodate specific symptoms and changes in phases of the disease. In the milder state of ARC (AIDS-related complex), therapy will vary from that of full-blown AIDS.

Many pioneers contribute to the advancement of herbal therapy for AIDS. Notables include Michael Young, author of "Chinese Herbal Therapies and HIV Infections: A Clinical Report," Makima Hawkins et al., "The Use of a Chinese Herbal Composition for the Treatment of HIV Infection," and Misha Cohen, "Acupuncture, AIDS, and Natural Healing," who recommends combination therapies, and Mary Kay Ryan and Arthur Shattuck, co-authors of *Treating AIDS with Chinese Medicine*.

Who treats AIDS patients with herbs?

Herbalists and acupuncturists in several cities care for AIDS patients. The Institute for Traditional Medicine maintains a current referral list with qualifications for anyone in need of a practitioner.

What is the prognosis for AIDS patients treated with acupuncture and herbs?

Under my care, AIDS patients have responded fairly well. I check symptoms, treat acupuncture points and dispense herbs, following suggestions from the researchers. Reduced complaints please both the patient and me. I have a very diversified practice to correct a multitude of disorders. So every favorable outcome satisfies me as a practitioner of Oriental medicine.

Acupuncture attempts to cure diseases by restoration of energy and removal of ills. Sometimes we fall short of complete remissions and can only relieve symptoms, which does help the patient. I feel we will attain the cure when we discover the right set of points, the right combination of herbs and the right Yin-Yang balanced life style.

A cannot-help-but-notice observation sticks out from worldwide fact-gathering projects: HIV appears less frequently in the Orient. Since our ratio of AIDS to population far exceeds that in China and Japan, the majority of case studies describe American patients.

Another remarkable observation concerns low rates of infection in China's hospitals and out-patient clinics. Without sterile disposable supplies and with sanitation way below standards in the United States, they still face fewer infected patients. Returning doctors from symposiums in Chinese medical institutions express their shock at the lack of shiny, clean, modern facilities, but also their astonishment at the fact that there are no infections.

In my opinion, exposure to the Chinese way of medical practice strengthens your energies, toughens your defenses, and increases your chances of survival. Oriental citizens commonly accept acupuncture and herbs as primary health care services in every stage of their lives. Even over-the-counter medications consist of natural ingredients, not manufactured chemicals. Breathing exercises, acupressure, needles, herbs, accommodations to seasonal change, all enhance disease prevention.

8

Cancer

Western medicine and Chinese medicine do not see eye to eye on cancer. The former tries to kill malignant cells to cure the disease. The latter, as it does with all sicknesses, normalizes energy to treat each symptom with efforts to prolong life. Thus most cancers in China get treated with acupuncture and herbs, not radiation and chemotherapy. Even in China, however, for localized tumors, surgeons often will perform excisions—under acupuncture anesthesia.

What is the actual difference between the Chinese and Western understandings of cancer?

The Latin root of the word "malignant" is *malus* and means maliciousness. So, in dealing with malignant tumors, Western medical thinking confronts enemy troops that multiply and spread malicious behavior. These conquering intruders attack the "innocent," healthy cells by unchecked reproduction with a plan to outnumber them.

Resorting to military strategy, Western medicine maneuvers for defense and counterattack. Weaponry consists of radiation and chemical warfare—chemotherapy. Repeated bombardment attempts to destroy the aggressor.

To grasp the Chinese perspective, in contrast, imagine a pure, fresh-water river, which runs with the same currents year after year. Suddenly, a large heavy object falls in and, by chance, forms a dam. A new waterway redirects the river from behind the obstruction. Meanwhile, in front of the barrier, water stagnates and soon turns into a thick swampy pool of hot decaying matter. The more the standing water shrinks, the more irregular, undesirable vegetation grows and accumulates. By analogy, Qi and Blood are like water, and Damp (with a physical growth) is like the unwanted vegetation. As Qi and Blood stagnate, and Damp gathers within the energy field, tumors grow in the body.

In acupuncture language, what is the disease process involved in cancer?

A long series of events precedes the actual formation of tumors. Stagnation of Qi is the principle cause. But the cause of this is Liver, which, if it is functioning poorly will fail to do its job of spreading energy. When Qi stagnates, Blood congeals and lumps form. To complicate matters, Damp collects because the Spleen cannot perform the duty of causing drying. Poison Fire settles with the accumulation. In general, the weakness of Qi and Blood lets the disease grow worse. All of this may be set in motion by excessive negative emotions.

Do acupuncturists evaluate and treat cancer with different concepts and methods from other diseases?

No, the same concepts and methods are applied to all diseases. In Chinese medicine, cancer is not identified as a disease as such. Symptoms which Western Medicine calls cancer are considered to be the result of dysfunctional Organs and damaging disruptions to the natural flow of Qi and Blood. The goal of acupuncture and Chinese herbology in general is to return the patient's Qi and Blood to normal. The symptoms of cancer are no exception. If complete return to normal proves impossible, we improve the body as much as possible. Relief of symptoms and the promotion of longevity are the direct motivations for all treatments. For these reasons, the indicated procedures for *every* disorder resemble each other.

What are the therapeutic actions of Chinese medicine in the case of cancer?

Since abnormal changes advance with a combination of factors, acupuncture and herbs attend to the individual details of the pathology. Needle insertion, often with moxa, circulates fresh Qi and Blood. We focus on breaking up stagnation (congealed Blood, Damp, Fire) and building up the immunity. Treatments are geared to both local tumors and systemic disharmonies, which must identify connected Organs.

Herbal formulas supplement needling and heat techniques. This combination adds significant benefits. From nature's backyard, a group of products strengthen the Qi and thereby strengthen the immune system. By means of an action called "blood cracking," congealed Blood dissipates and debris exits to permit healing.

Research conducted over the centuries informs us of the various effects of ingesting plants and animal parts. For example, the cleansing of toxins curtails tumor growth after the ingestion of certain leaves and flowers. Animal cartilage also interferes with cancers. A favorite concoction is shark fin soup, which has been around as a tonic for generations. To soften masses, we use minerals from the shells of sea animals. Anticancer substances arrive from diverse sources, unfortunately not all of which are available in the United States. In China, to fulfill the requirements of Oriental health practices, pharmacies in every province are skilled in the preparation of medicines from crude herbs.

What types of cancers can acupuncture treat?

In Chinese medical literature, we find specific needle points and herbs indicated for specific disharmonies and the tumors. Disharmonies listed relate to cancer of the bone, brain, breast, cervix, esophagus, gallbladder, liver, lung, nose, pancreas, pharynx, prostate, stomach, uterus, Hodgkin's disease, and leukemia.

Does acupuncture really cure cancer?

In the early stages, before the occurrence of massive tumors, cures are possible. Unlike radiation and chemotherapy, Chinese methods try to keep the person strong and otherwise healthy. But even in the presence of a growth, the direction of care is to eradicate symptoms, lengthen life, maintain the unaffected cells as best as possible, and hopefully to cure the affliction.

Can acupuncture do anything for patients undergoing Western chemotherapy by way of relieving side-effects such as fatigue, nausea, and hair loss?

Certainly. An acupuncturist will select applications with needles and herbs to reduce your complaints and give you strength.

The rapid increase of cases of cancer seems to be fairly recent. Western scientific cancer research also is relatively new. How can an ancient form of medicine treat such a contemporary crises as this disease?

It is true that an age-old practice of medicine preserves principles of diagnosis and therapy, century after century, millennium after millennium. Countless generations have recovered when faced with all kinds of sickness. Acupuncture applies eternal facts of nature to any disharmony of life.

Historical documentation permits us to study and use methods from the past. For instance, horrendous plagues hit China around the year 200 C.E., which resembled the European plagues of the Middle Ages. We read how Chinese victims were treated by applying the identical basic concepts still in practice today. We thus should be encouraged to apply similar care to modern life-threatening epidemics. Though physical diagnostic terms usually change through the ages, Qi, Blood and Organs stay the same. Also unchanged is the prescription of needle points and herbs.

Where are the sources for the herbs in their raw state?

Many natural products are used in preparing medication for cancer. Natural herbs are harvested and processed like food, because they *are* food. Crude herbs grow, for instance, as roots, mushrooms, fruits, leaves, tubers, bark, flowers, spurs, resins, bulbs, seeds, plant tops, whole plants, animal shells and antlers, and wasp nests. I guess the maxim "seek and you shall find" applies to the Chinese search for the most medicinal substances provided by nature.

9

Neurological and Emotional Disturbances

How are emotions related to the organs?

The Chinese correlate disease origins to emotional problems based on Organ energy. Prolonged agitation disturbs Qi. On the other hand, an Organ dysfunction can give rise to troubled feelings.

How can I control or prevent self-destructive emotions?

Many forms of Meditation, Yoga, as well as the Chinese body and breathing exercises of Tai Chi Chuan and Qigong all generate inner strength, inner peace, and inner health. These practices can help you contact the healing Qi energy within you. Choose a method that you feel attracted to, practice it with a sincere appreciation for the blessings you are receiving, and integrate it into your life in a harmonious way. Certainly, acupuncture can help balance energy to avert feelings that tear you apart. Over my many years as an acupuncturist I have noticed wonderful responses from patients who practice the energetic arts such as Yoga. Their awareness of their own Qi energy frequently develops to the point where they feel acupuncture healing taking place instantly.

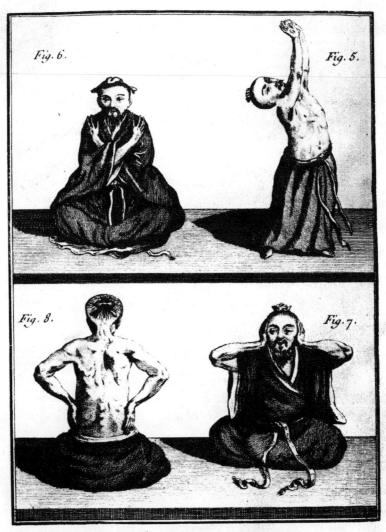

Traditional Chinese "Qigong" (energy exercise) positions

How does acupuncture relate emotions to the nervous system?

Neurological diseases like multiple sclerosis, neuropathy, Parkinson's, Bell's palsy, and paralysis are serious physical disorders; nevertheless, in the West when we say we're "nervous" we are not necessarily refering to defects in our physical nervous system. Physically a nerve is a tissue, but the word also denotes courage, vigor, and even audacity. In this way our language actually reflects an attitude that is quite in conformity with acupuncture principles, which see objective physiology and subjective, psychological qualities as essentially one. But in practice, Western medical science emphasizes objective physiology and puts emotion, sensation, and inner attitude in the category of psychology, not physical medicine.

In this way, Western medicine has created in-depth experiments to uncover the mechanisms behind impulses, secretions, and the transmission of neurological signals; we understand the junctions of nervous tissue with muscles, the origins of the sensations of touch and the other senses, and the structure of the spinal cord, and scientists are learning more about the functioning of the brain every research day. Neurology embraces the anatomy and biochemistry of nerves. We understand the role played by electricity in the nervous system, and this in turn helps us understand nerve fiber activity.

Acupuncture sees all these phenomena from a different perspective and perceives Qi energy as the principle working within sensation and bodily movement. Qi thus guides all nerve functioning, but it also is operative in our subjective sensations and emotional feelings as well. This is why for the acupuncturist your emotions and precise sensations are as important as what is occurring within you physiologically. But this does not mean that what Western medicine considers physical factors are ignored. Neurological disability in the back or limbs will mean impairment to the Channels, perhaps from direct injury. Channel energy travels roughly in parallel with the nerves, along the spine and through the brain. Knowledge of physiological problems can thus give clues as to blockages in the flow of Qi energy.

Can acupuncture treat multiple sclerosis?

The most common symptom of MS is weakening limbs. In Western terms, the Central Nervous System shows dispersed patches on the myelin sheathes that form coverings around the brain and spinal cord.

Acupuncture treatment for MS focuses on Organ energy and Channels that run beside the vertebrae. Generally, in MS a harmful inside-body climate accompanies stagnation of Blood and Qi. Since MS rarely strikes anyone in China, it took a while for acupuncturists to understand the pathology in acupuncture terms. Now we know that an initial Heat in the Lungs leads to deficiencies of the Kidney and Liver.

Needling will drain injurious substances, perhaps Damp and Heat, and invite healthy energy and Blood. The demyelinated nerves need nourishment provided by therapy. Acupuncture also shifts energy from the interior to the exterior or from one side to the other.

You may experience results immediately or over a long term of therapy. Different people respond in different ways. One of my patients regained full use of an arm after the first treatment. The legs improved slowly with limitation. I feel that everybody with multiple sclerosis should try acupuncture.

What causes the shaking in Parkinson's disease?

Wind in the Channels, aroused by a Liver energy disorder, causes the tremors. This is treatable by regulating the Liver, Yin and Yang imbalances, and Qi and Blood circulation.

What Organs ordinarily cause nervous and mental disorders?

The Heart, Pericardium, and Liver.

How does acupuncture treat addiction to smoking, drugs, alcoholism, and overeating?

Acupuncture has achieved noted successes in curbing specific abnormal cravings. Addiction is actually a multifaceted issue. Needle point stimulation can be very useful combined with sessions with psychologists or with group therapy, particularly for drugs and alcohol.

The most commonly used points in cases of addiction are in the ear. These points are thought to have direct connections to the brain. Precise needling techniques break the addiction, relax the person, strengthen the emotions and replace internal feelings of *emptiness* that may be at the root of the addiction.

Each kind of obsession may present subsidiary problems. For instance, frequently Lung disorders accompany smoking. Asthma, bronchitis, emphysema, pneumonia, therefore, must also receive treatment. Overweight, obviously, may accompany overeating, problems in food absorption and fluid retention. It therefore justifies improvement of the digestive Organs or the elimination of excess Damp.

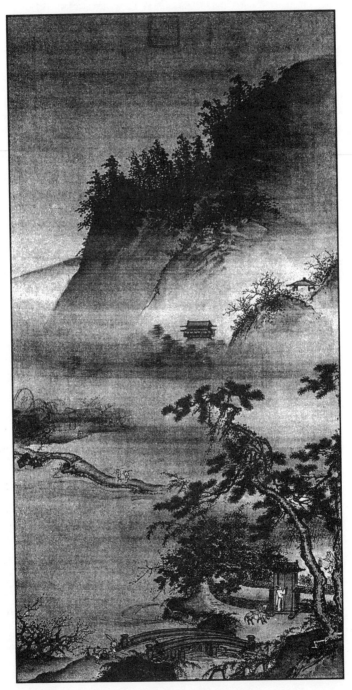

Tai Chin, Returning Late from Spring Outing
(Ca. 1440)

10

Case Studies

Sciatica

A middle-aged woman named Ann made an appointment in my office for what she said was an inflammation of her sciatic nerve, diagnosed as sciatica. Ann was a cheerful, heavy sort, who described a burning soreness in back of her thigh and pain around her hip and waist. Due to poor control of urination, she had undergone bladder surgery, which unfortunately did not help. Another complaint concerned a searing discomfort of the ovaries before each menstrual cycle. Also an ovarian cyst developed. Other than chiropractic adjustments to relieve the hip pain periodically, no doctor could offer a clear explanation of her problems.

I examined her tongue, which showed an internal presence of harmful Heat. The pulses sent a message of deficient energy for urinary and reproductive Organs. A few treatments released the trapped Heat and toughened Urinary Bladder and Kidney energy. Afterwards, Ann reported no more burning of her ovary, no more hip pain and stronger urinary functions. The really good news was that an ultrasound examination revealed the complete disappearance of the ovarian cyst. To correct Ann's problem, I had to evaluate disturbances and improve the flow of energy encircling the waist.

Multiple Disorders

Carl, a twenty-seven year old, active, single man, complained of knee pain and weakness. Damp weather aggravated his knees. In addition, breathing difficulties arose from allergies to dairy products. Also, he had trouble falling asleep and suffered from prostatitis, even at his young age. Since Western medicine views Carl as having four unrelated disorders, he sought help with specialists who treat different parts of the body. His consultants included an allergist, orthopedic surgeon, and urologist. Knee surgery was recommended, a lactose-free diet kept allergies in check, and, for awhile, antibiotics treated the inflamed prostate. No suggestions came forth for the insomnia.

As an acupuncturist, I sought connections between the ailments. Tongue examination showed some Yang Heat of the Heart and a generally Damp interior. This fired-up Heat of the Heart accounted for his insomnia. Heat from the Heart can fall into the Small Intestine and cause certain types of urologic inflammation. The Heart and Small Intestine are Yin-Yang partners and the Small Intestine deals with urinary functions. At this point I partly knew the reason for the prostate problem. The Heart-related sleeplessness became clear, as did Dampness on the knees. Exterior moisture will further disrupt wetness inside.

The pulse gave me readings of a rapid Heart and deficient Spleen, Lung and Kidney. Using the Five Element Cycle, I understood that an obstacle blocked the Qi between the Heart and the Spleen. In turn, the Organs following the Spleen in the cyclic pattern (the Lung and Kidney) were also cut off from sufficient supplies of Qi. Now all the symptoms had a place. The weakened Spleen could not fully carry out its work to move moisture and transform food. Moist milk, not metabolized, burdened an already deficient Lung, to cause allergic reactions in breathing. Reduced Kidney Qi contributed to the prostatitis and played the culprit for painful, weak knees.

I directed Carl's treatment toward a rehabilitation of energy flow by following the Generating Cycle. *(See the chart on page 50).*

Opening the Heart-Spleen barrier regulated Heart excess and allowed Qi to gush into the Spleen, Lung and Kidney. Points to manipulate energy for general restoration received supplements for local relief of symptoms. I inserted needles on all four limbs, the chest, abdomen and back. A series of office visits brought Carl correction of his ailments.

Dental Problem

An example of diverse methods well-integrated within a single profession is to be found in dentistry. Dental practitioners make use of X ray, surgery, drugs, mechanics, nutrition, the natural care of gum massage, herbal remedies, and a growing application of acupuncture. Micro-acupuncture systems found in the mouth include tongue diagnostic patterns. Points on the ear, hand and foot offer analgesia and regulating therapies for tooth problems. I've gotten good results for TMJ (temporal mandibular joint) problems with facial techniques. As in every field of health, acupuncture will fill many needs.

A registered nurse named Sandy felt tenderness in a molar following much corrective dentistry. Denuded bone had left the underlying tissue and nerve exposed. She asked me if acupuncture could generate new bone to avoid a surgery that transplants bone from the opposite jaw area. I explained how Kidney energy controls bone and how, by needling, Qi and Blood enters disturbed body parts to nourish and heal. We then went to work.

Points and methods I selected strengthened Kidney Qi and motivated Qi and Blood to circulate through the jaw. Congestive blocks drained out with other needle stick approaches. Gradually, Sandy noticed less and less discomfort in her tooth. After a series of treatments, her dentist took X rays. To the delight of us all, new bone had formed to fill the vacant spot. The transplant surgery was not necessary.

Kidney Stones

A thirty-five year old man came to me for a vexing case of kidney stones. He suffered from burning in the kidneys, low back pain, frequent urination, and ringing in the ears. After he told me of his two surgeries for spleen and gallbladder removal, he said "no more surgery." Pulse examination informed me of abnormal Spleen, Liver, Gallbladder and Urinary Bladder. (Even though the physical aspect of an Organ is absent after surgery, its energy remains.) Studying the moisture on the tongue's red body, I knew there was a presence of Damp Heat.

An assessment of this man informed me that his Spleen Qi and Liver Qi had been disturbed. As a result, the internal environment lacked the ability to dry excess dampness and disperse congested areas. Stagnation can eventually manifest Heat, which in fact developed here. Weakness also hurt the urinary system.

Damp Heat produces kidney stones. How this happens can be understood by analogy. Just as *wet* clay becomes hard dry pottery in a *hot* kiln, or *moist* dough solidifies into bread when *baked* in an oven, kidney stones form from *Damp* Heat. The way to cure this disease, therefore, is to get rid of the Damp and the Heat.

I chose points to restore the Spleen's moisture-drying ability. Other points cooled down and drained the Fire. It was vital to bring back the normalcy of the urinary system through Kidney rehabilitation. My goals in treatment also included dispersion of congestion.

When I first inserted the needles, the patient expressed immediate relief. Several office visits later (the series of treatments lasted through the summer, autumn and winter months), the symptoms finally disappeared. No more burning, no more pains, no more frequent urination, and no more ringing in the ears. Together, these improvements reflected no more Damp Heat, no more Kidney deficiency and no more kidney stones.

One of the most pleasing outcomes concerned the patient's wife's cooking. Previously, many of her dishes aggravated his symptoms. This greatly limited his diet. Now he can eat anything she prepares.

High Blood Sugar

Nancy, a massage therapist, complained of numbness at her fingertips. A physical exam discovered high blood sugar. Where Western medicine would have connected the two problems as indicating diabetic neuropathy (nerve disturbance associated with diabetes), I found a Kidney deficiency. A weak Kidney pulse informed me of this. The patient's history of a hypothyroid condition and cravings for salt indicated an Organ downslide as well. I matched the lack of finger sensation with the Triple Burner Channel. This makes sense since the Lower Burner relates to the Kidney and the Triple Burner Channel terminates in the afflicted fingers.

I selected points to regulate the Kidney and promote the secretion of insulin by the pancreas. There are pancreas points in addition to those for the combined Spleen-Pancreas Organ. By self-testing, the patient watched a fall in blood sugar. Then, with help from the heat of moxibustion, normal feelings returned to the fingers.

Chronic Constipation

An eight year-old girl, highly intelligent and studious, came to my office with her parents, to seek help for chronic constipation. What was diagnosed as uncontrolled elimination at four and a half had become irregularity three years later. X-ray examination illustrated an enlarged and full colon. The hospital doctor who cared for the child recommended a year of drinking mineral oil. Concerned about ill effects and nutritional impairment from a petroleum based liquid, more natural and less risky methods were considered such as acupuncture.

My examination of the pulses and tongue showed a very weak Large Intestine. The Large Intestine pulse was actually empty. It only took four treatments to normalize the colon and correct the problem. I was able to detect changes with the touch of my finger as the pulse re-energized itself.

Bellyache

On a Friday afternoon, A twelve year old girl with a bloated, painful abdomen came into the office with her mother. The mother was fearful of surgical exploration, if they went to the hospital. A few years earlier, the daughter had undergone an appendectomy, but now, once again, had symptoms similar to appendicitis. The symptoms were no appetite, sore throat, fever, and aggravation of pain on manual pressure to the hardened lower abdomen. This meant the presence of Intestinal Abscess. Chinese medicine calls it Stagnation of Blood and Heat in the Large Intestine. Tongue and pulse examinations confirmed the diagnosis. This correlates with appendicitis in Western medicine; however, without the appendix, the harmful, internal condition still persisted.

Within an hour, I had drained the Heat and cleared the Stagnant Blood. Acupuncture needling also regulated Large Intestine Qi and promoted some Yin. The mother sat next to her lying-ever-so-still daughter and saw the miraculous changes take place. Immediate fever reduction followed flattening of the swollen abdomen, elimination of the sore throat and return of normal complexion. The daughter felt total relief and returned to school on the following Monday.

Dislocated Shoulder

Sports medicine today is an ever-growing practice, with specializations emerging for every kind of competition. "Javelin shoulder," "tennis elbow," and "baseball finger" are part of the vocabulary of their respective games. Although I treat several forms of injury experienced by athletes in a variety of sports, my most frequent patients are tennis players. (In fact,the tennis coach of a university in my area unofficially designated me team acupuncturist.)

One referral came to me with a painful shoulder and a history of a dislocated shoulder blade. An MRI showed soft tissue damage. To engage in the sport, this student had to have her underarm thoroughly taped. Unable to tolerate the pain caused by the injured tissue, she compensated by using other muscles. Hitting the ball became an ordeal.

Questions, examination, and tongue diagnosis confirmed a Cold blockage in Channels that pass through the arm. Acupuncture cleared the Channels, strengthened the muscles, and supported the bones. With the additional heat of moxa, tennis practice resumed as normal after a few days. Not only did acupuncture relieve all pain and restore function, but the shoulder blade moved back into place.

AIDS

A thirty-five year old male with AIDS sought help for problems of fatigue and neuropathy of the arms and legs. The nerve disorder of neuropathy displayed symptoms of pain and weakness. Other ailments were sinus conditions, respiration and digestion difficulties, dizziness, ringing in the ear, muffled hearing and emotional depression. Obviously, disturbances affected the Three Burners and extremity Channels.

Because of the HIV-positive state, I emphasized the rehabilitation of immunity. Needles, herbal medication, and moxa enhanced the Qi, Blood and Essence, while poisons drained from the body's interior. Complaints subsided after I energized the upper and lower limbs and regulated the Lung, Stomach and Kidney. Acupuncture did not cure the AIDS, but it brought symptom relief, strength and better feelings.

Tumors

A woman I had been treating for menopausal symptoms discovered a tumor on her breast. She wished not to undergo any surgical procedure, including biopsy. She wanted to resolve the growth in an easy and natural way.

I selected acupuncture points, which influence the Liver to spread Qi, and which clear the Channels passing through the breast. Dispersement of stagnation was a major consideration. From the Kidneys, I took assistance to fortify the Liver.

The tumor shrank smaller and smaller after each consecutive visit. After four treatments, it disappeared and never returned. We do not know whether the lesion was malignant or benign, since the pathological tissue was never examined in the laboratory. Of course, Qi Energy can only be evaluated on the live individual. It really doesn't matter if we learned the status of abnormal cells, for in the long run we got rid of the stagnating Qi, the Channel blockage, and the breast tumor.

Multiple Disorders

Regularly, I suggest that patients jot down particulars about how they feel between visits. These notes should include descriptions of physical and emotional experiences. Sometimes a person greets me with pages filled with exact locations of discomfort, functional problems, and psychological illustrations. All this is very helpful, and, as we make progress, hopefully there's less to write about.

One wife and mother in the full-time work force used to outline her condition on paper. In fine detail, she depicted where pain existed, what needed increases and what needed elimination. Evaluation of the many complaints and desires showed that everything had a place. Symptoms were: circles under the eyes, the urge to urinate too frequently, the want of joy and enthusiasm, pain below the naval, hope for improvement in memory, in concentration and in vocalization, craving better sexual and spiritual energy, tension in the back. Taken together these symptoms targeted Kidney and related Heart disharmonies. Multiple symptoms revealed the intricacy of the involvement of other Organs and various Channels.

After weeks of therapy, the flood of disorders trickled down to a few, then nothing. The patient got off her medications and literally put life back into her living.

Bibliography

Suggested General Reading

Beinfeld, Harriet and Korngold, Efrem. *Between Heaven and Earth: A Guide To Chinese Medicine*, (New York: Ballantine Books, 1991).

Byers, Dwight. *Better Health with Foot Reflexology*, (Saint Petersburg, Florida: Ingham Publishing, Inc., 1983).

Bloomfield, Frena. *The Book of Chinese Beliefs*, (London: Arrow Books Limited, 1983).

Clayre, Alasdair. *The Heart of the Dragon*, (Boston: Houghton Mifflin Company, 1986).

Connelly, Dianne. *Traditional Acupuncture: the Law of the Five Elements*, (Columbia, Maryland: The Center For Traditional Acupuncture, 1979).

Cooper, J. C. *Chinese Alchemy*, (New York: Sterling Publishing Company Inc., 1990).

Dale, Ralph Alan. *The Origins and Future of Acupuncture*, (North Miami Beach, Florida: Dialectic Publishing, Inc., 1982).

Hammer, Leon. *Dragon Rises, Red Bird Flies*, (Barrytown, New York: Station Hill Press, 1990).

Kaptchuck, Ted. *The Web That Has No Weaver*, (New York: Congdon & Weed, Inc., 1983).

Lu, Henry. *Chinese System of Food Cures*, (New York: Sterling Publishing Company Inc., 1986).

Mann, Felix. *Acupuncture the Ancient Art of Healing and How It Works Scientifically*, (New York: Vintage Books, 1973).

Reid, Daniel. *Chinese Herbal Medicine*, (Boston: Shambhala Publications Inc., 1993).

Suggested Professional Reading

Bensky, Dan and O'Connor, John. *Acupuncture, A Comprehensive Text*, (Chicago: Eastland Press, 1983).

Bensky, Dan and Gamble, Andrew. *Chinese Herbal Medicine Materia Medica*, (Seattle, Washington: Eastland Press, 1993).

Birch, Stephen and Matsumoto, Kiiko. *Five Elements and Ten Stems*, (Higganum, Connecticut: Paradigm Publications, no date).

Chen, Xinnong et al. *Chinese Acupuncture and Moxibustion*, (Beijing: Foreign Language Press, 1990).*

Dale, Ralph Alan. *Dictionary of Acupuncture*, (North Miami Beach, Florida: Dialectic Publishing, Inc., 1993).

Dharmananda, Subhuti. *Chinese Herbal Therapies for Immune Disorders*, (Portland, Oregon: Institute For Traditional Medicine, 1991).

Jirui, Chen and Wang, Nissi. *Acupuncture Case Histories from China*, (Seattle, Washington: Eastland Press, 1988).

Lade, Arne. *Acupuncture Points Images & Functions*, (Seattle, Washington: Eastland Press, 1989).

Low, Royston. *The Secondary Vessels of Acupuncture*, (New York: Thorson Publishers Inc., 1985).

Maciocia, Giovanni. *Tongue Diagnosis in Chinese Medicine*, (Seattle, Washington: Eastland Press, 1987).

Porkert, Manfred. *The Theoretical Foundations of Chinese Medicine*, (Cambridge, Massachusetts: The MIT Press, 1985).

Ryan, Mary Kay and Shattuck, Arthur. *Treating AIDS with Chinese Medicine*, (Berkeley, California: Pacific View Press, 1994).

Scott, Julian. *Acupuncture in the Treatment of Children*, (Seattle, Washington: Eastland Press, 1991).

So, James Tin Yau. *Treatment of Disease with Acupuncture*, (Brookline, Massachusetts: Paradigm Publications, 1987).

Woollerton, Henry and McLean, Colleen. *Acupuncture Energy in Health and Disease*, (Wellingborough, Northamptonshire, Great Britain: Thorson Publishers Limited, 1986).

Zhen, Li Shi. *Pulse Diagnosis*, (Brookline, Massachusetts: Paradigm Publications, 1985).

Zhu, Mingqing. A *Handbook for Treatment of Acute Syndromes by Using Acupuncture and Moxibustion*, (Hong Kong: 8 Dragon Publishing, 1991).

Chinese Acupuncture and Moxibustion is a revision of *Essentials of Chinese Acupuncture*

Index